A Nursing School Diary

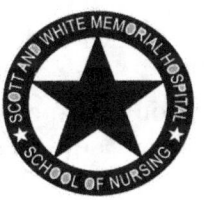

By

Norma Hammond Mc Loughlin RN

2010

Mc Loughlin Publishers
155 Rush Haven Dr.,
The Woodlands, Tx. 77381-3032

281 367 3147

mclou@hal-pc.org
jnmclou@gmail.com

Introduction

On a whim I began writing daily notes in a diary when I started nursing school on September 5, 1954. With no plans for the contents, other than my own memories, the book was stored away. Twenty-five years later, while planning for our class reunion, I had an idea that I could use the old diary to write a short history of our experiences on the bumpy road to becoming registered nurses. Sorting through the pages, I chose entries that were particularly interesting—incidents and events that my classmates might recall with fondness and nostalgia (or in some cases prefer not to recall at all). The result was this slightly expurgated, but true, narrative of the lives of the class of 1957

Now that another twenty-five years have passed, it occurred to me that by publishing the book other RN's from our generation might find it fun to read and compare with their own recollections. In this day and age of coed dorms and broad-minded lifestyles, more recent nursing school graduates will be amused, or downright amazed at the restrictions we accepted on our personal lives and the enormous changes that have come about in nursing education in the ensuing years

We looked like "angels of mercy" in our stiff white uniforms. The winged sides on the white cap added to the illusion. And, all of us fell in love with that image. In the hospital, everyone tried for perfection. About half of our small class led a squeaky clean existence

24/7. The rest of us managed to find entertainment in our off hours that wasn't Florence-Nightingale approved. In fact, had we been discovered, I'm sure "She" would have disowned us.

Despite our differences, we became very close—probably more like sisters than those linked by genetic ties. For more than fifty years our class has met for a reunion every two to three years. We married, had children, moved to far flung locations (some to other countries), but we never lost touch with each other.

With the exception of one classmate who became a teacher, we all stayed in the nursing profession. One became a nurse anesthetist, one worked in a doctor's office, one in psychiatry, one in public health, one in obstetrics, two in home health, one in hospice care, three worked in varied hospital and clinic settings, and I worked as a school nurse.

Over the years most of us tried several different areas of nursing. Our extensive clinical experience in nursing school made the transitions easy. My own history included: medical/surgical bedside nursing at Methodist Hospital in Dallas, oncology at Gaston Hospital in Dallas, emergency room at West Suburban Hospital in Chicago, recovery room and ICU at Ochsner Hospital in New Orleans, operating room at West Jefferson Hospital in Marrero, Louisiana, sixteen years as a school nurse at St. Martin's Episcopal School in Metairie, Louisiana, and a six year stint in neonatology at Memorial Hermann Hospital in The Woodlands, Texas.

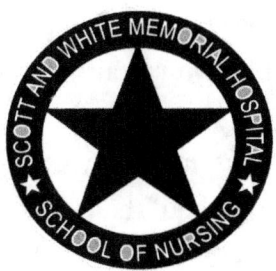

How did we know where to assemble? Did someone send instructions? Somehow we all managed to be moving into our new home on September 1, 1954. There was much confusion as parents deposited eighteen scared, but excited, girls in "Senior Dormitory" on the Scott and White campus. (Well—seventeen anyway—I was the only one to arrive by train—alone—carrying all my earthly belongings in one suitcase.)

Roommates were pre-assigned. Mine (Jackie) spent the first evening filling the small closet in our room with what seemed to be hundreds of outfits. I told her not to worry—that I only had one dress anyway! I sat on the bed and watched—in awe. It was apparent from that auspicious beginning that we had nothing in common.

Exploring the facilities didn't take long. The majority of us would be living on the second floor in double occupancy rooms (one room on each floor was a single). Each room was furnished with twin beds, a dresser, desk, chair, and a goose-neck desk lamp. A bathroom was at the end of the upstairs hall. A single shower, commode, and lavatory were to accommodate the thirteen of us living

on that floor. The phone was midway of the hall (the number—
PR8-8667). A large porch at the end of the hallway seemed to
slope precariously. It was closed in at the bottom half, with screen
the rest of the way up. Downstairs a sitting room was furnished
with a well-used sofa, several chairs, and an upright piano. Doro-
thy Anderson (our housemother) was already ensconced in a fairly
large bedroom to the right of the front entrance. The stairwell
occupied a substantial portion of the downstairs area, but there were
three student rooms at the back. The bath on that floor sported a
claw-foot bathtub to go with the one lavatory and commode. There
was also a phone in the downstairs hallway. The front door opened
onto a generous porch with a porch swing at each end.

We were up bright and early the next morning for physical exams.
A nurse, who appeared to have been dipped in starch, was in charge
of student health. Dr. Fred Hammond was the student health doctor. What an interesting group we must have been. They kept us
all day in the clinic.

Poor Dr. Hammond. I'm sure he didn't deserve it, but Dottie immediately dubbed him "Lacy Drawers."

On September 3rd we dutifully filled our urine specimen bottles
and carted them over to the hospital. If this was our first assignment, we seem to have passed the test. We were given the rest of
the day off. Joyce Lott and I walked downtown, looked in all the
shops, and treated ourselves to banana splits. Actually, there aren't
many shops in town. It's a sleepy little burg, but I can already tell
that I love it.

Apparently they're serious! We're truly student nurses! Our first books were passed out in Classroom I this morning. This $26.56 purchase felt like a major step. The heft of those books generated quite a bit of pride.

Our "big sisters" took Dottie and me out on the town to introduce us to the night life. We visited the U.S.O. (where there were more young men than I had ever seen in one building), then to the Shangri-La. It was Saturday night, so we could stay out until midnight, and we took full advantage.

Our first S&W social function was a sunrise breakfast at a nearby park "early" on Sunday morning. No sun appeared, and the sky was overcast with dark clouds—matching our ungrateful faces.

Alarm clocks went off all over the dorm at six o'clock on Monday morning. Now the rubber will meet the road! We marched over to the classrooms, after dutifully eating our cafeteria breakfast, and met all of the faculty. Quite an impressive assemblage! Did any of us think we would ever look like Miss Broughton—the epitome of professional nursing? (I suspected she even ironed her shoelaces.) Our only requirement for the day seemed to be a personality test. Perhaps they didn't want to overload us until they checked out our psyches. Come to think of it—maybe they sent Johnie Johnson as a part of the test. She joined our class that evening. It was like suddenly finding an exotic bird in the midst of a barnyard full of chicks. None of us knew quite what to make of her.

Another day in Classroom #1 spent on getting acquainted. Johnie was formally introduced to the class.

On September 8th a big yellow bus picked us up at the dorm and conveyed us to Temple Junior College. Sat through two classes and a lecture. The bus ride was the high point of the day. We sang most of the trip—both ways. We're beginning to bond!

That week-end I convinced Lou to join my date (no doubt someone I met at the Shangri-La), his friend, and me. We drove to Fort Hood. It was my first football game, and Lou's first date. (Two catastrophes for the price of one!)

On September 13th we met our new anatomy lecturer—a young man with piercing eyes, red hair, and a surly attitude. He talked faster than we could write. On our walk back to the dorm after class, we all agreed that we would never learn anything from Dr. Daniels. His favorite expression was "church is out," and we were beginning to feel that we might be part of that congregation.

To divert us from too much misery and introspection, we were treated to a picnic at Scott and White Dairy Farm. Food being the second or third item on our priority list—it probably worked.

We were given a long list of rules to live by. The strangest of the lot was that we couldn't walk on the hospital side of the street nor go anywhere on the hospital campus wearing pants. Getting in a car wearing shorts was also forbidden.

Curfew was at eight o'clock on week-nights, midnight on Friday and Saturday, and ten o'clock on Sunday. Staying out past curfew could bring punishment—anywhere from being "campused" for a few minutes violation to expulsion if deemed excessive enough. We learned to be on the porch on time—even if we didn't rush in. The porch swings were often filled with couples saying good night.

Those who lingered too long were given a not too subtle warning by Andy that she was locking the door shortly—with us in—or out. If we wanted to stay out later than curfew on a week-end, there was something called "overnight permission." We were required to ask (in writing) ahead of time and have it approved by Miss Cole or her designate (usually Miss Gallman). This was necessary even if we were going home for the weekend. We soon found though that we could sign out to stay at a classmate's home. Mr. and Mrs. Stroud must have cursed the rule, since they often found extra girls in Dottie's bed and around their breakfast table on Sunday mornings.

I don't know that it was ever an edict from Miss Cole that we couldn't go to any of the nightclubs except the Shangri-La, Tally Ho, and the Idle Hour. I doubt she would have admitted she knew where they were. Upperclassmen let us know that we would be in serious trouble if we were caught in the seamier places. (Obviously we thought the key word was "caught".) The more adventurous of our group (a.k.a. the bad seeds) couldn't resist the live bands and even livelier crowds at the Royal Club, the S&S, Park and Eat, Cascade, Catalina, Canteen, and the Sheep Shed Inn.

Rooms had to be kept neat and clean at all times. Walk through inspections were common. We were not to cook in the dormitory. Duh! We had no kitchen. (We did make some fairly decent meals in Peggy's popcorn popper though.) No men above the first floor (did that exempt Frenchie, Joni, Kathryn, Johnie, and Muriel, whose rooms were on the first floor, from the no men rule?). We rarely even had gentlemen callers in the sitting room anyway. We preferred it for ourselves. Most of our dates were met at the door.

We could starve the remainder of the day if so desired (fat chance!), but we were required to show up in the cafeteria and consume a full breakfast (apparently to keep our strength up for the day's activities).

Gladys was the regular maid for our dorm—a more motherly soul couldn't be found--nor a better friend to a houseful of immature girls. She was always ready to lend a hand (or advice) if needed. And the infectious laughter that frequently rolled from her ample bosom could brighten the dreariest day. She scolded us for our transgressions, but never tattled. An alternate, Sallie Mae, wasn't quite in the same ball park with Gladys. We never would have trusted her with our secrets—in fact, she likely had a direct pipeline to Miss Cole. But, she was sort of fun—in a flighty sort of way. Their "required" duties only included cleaning the common areas, the bathrooms, and the floors.

Collins Janeway became a part of our lives. He owned the drugstore next to classrooms I and II. We soon discovered that everyone hung out there before, between, and after classes. We felt almost as much at home around the tables in the drugstore as we did in the dorm. He allowed all the students to run a tab if they wished, and pay at the end of the month—for cosmetics, supplies, magazines, food, etc. Only a few of our class, who knew their parents would bail them out, took advantage of his generosity. Most of us operated on a cash basis (as in—doing without until payday).

Our first pay day was on September 16th. We were so proud of that $7.50 check. Of course, most of us went out and spent it immediately. Prudence and frugality would come later!

September is almost over, and we've settled into a routine with classes and exams. We are taking five classes (Nursing Arts, Literature, Chemistry, Anatomy and Physiology, and Microbiology), and sometimes they all fall on one day. After the unit exam in Anatomy on Monday, we had all been convinced that we failed. When our grades came back it was a great relief—since I made 94, I'm sure that others did even better. We're smarter than we thought!

What a glorious spectacle—all of us dressed in starched white uniforms and borrowed caps—dazzling the crowd as we sang at a local fair. How strange it felt to wear the caps, even for that short period, when we were working so hard to earn our own.

Nursing Arts seems like a vacation following microbiology labs. We're torn between two opinions about Mrs. Newton, our micro instructor. She is either an obsessive compulsive psychotic—or just a nut that hates student nurses and fears germs (in that order). Either way, she plans to flunk us all, and totally humiliate us along the way.

On the other end of the spectrum—our chemistry professor (Mr. McCall) was as soft as mush. He had no idea how to handle a room full of girls, but he loved us anyway. The fact that he was well past retirement age probably gave us an added advantage. We were woefully inadequate in his class. Only Carol, Marjorie, and perhaps Joyce Helbert had a good background in chemistry. A few of the others actually seemed to know what he was talking about once in a while. We went through the motions in the labs and lectures, but some days resorted to singing to him for half the class, or getting him started on unrelated discussions that he often lost the battle to control.

Tonight Joyce Lott and I opted for a walk in the rain since we were bored and curfew was an hour away. (Actually, it was a storm with blowing wind and solid sheets of water.) We donned plastic raincoats over our shorty pajamas and sloshed our way around several blocks—confident that no one of importance would be out to see us, but feeling quite daring just the same.

On October 7th we were taken on a tour of the hospital—all dressed in our uniforms. They even let us explore some old rooms that contained outdated equipment. One machine had been used to bring up body heat to "kill" syphilis germs (before penicillin). There was also something called "the house of wax".

The "hospital" is actually a compound consisting of several buildings—each in its own unique architectural style. They are called Main building, West building, Clinic, Four and Five Cottages, and Cora Anderson Negro Hospital. Santa Fe Hospital, which isn't on this campus, is also operated by Scott and White.

We're learning to make up hospital beds in Nursing Arts class. The morning of October 12th we were graded on a "surgical bed". Miss Bohls, as always, seemed as nervous as we were. After class, Carol, Johnie, Sue, Ruthie, and I went downtown to see the movie, *Magnificent Obsession*. (We probably thought it was about us.)

Kathleen Barrington bailed out . She decided to get married instead of staying in school. We sang *Auld Lang Syne* to her on her last day riding the bus back from class. We all cried. Such hypocrites! We hardly knew her, and few of us had tried. She must have seemed ancient to us—she was around thirty.

Most of our clinical experience is on North and South End. We're getting to know Mrs. Pike and Miss Phleuger awfully well. One thing we've learned is that Mrs. Pike has no sense of humor. Nursing care is SERIOUS business! She made it quite clear that she eats student nurses for breakfast—and they aren't her favorite morsels. Miss Phleuger was a bit more approachable, and seemed not to mind our stupid questions.

I wouldn't have been surprised to be asked to mop the floor. We did everything else. Bed baths with complete care—brushing teeth, combing hair, and rubbing backs. Changing sheets and cleaning beds. Emptying bed pans, emesis basins, and Gomco suction and catheter bottles (praying each time that the hopper would flush without splashing). Cleaning the tops of those metal bedside tables with our little paper towels of comet cleanser until they were shining. Emptying the wastebaskets, and cleaning and filling the water pitchers. And even straightening up the patient's room, and caring for floral arrangements. In our "spare" time we folded newspapers to be used for wastebasket liners and cleaned thermometers and other equipment. I guess at this point in time we were only snappily dressed maids, but we felt important and had a lot of pride in our work.

Good thing we all had healthy egos. They were trampled daily as we waited for every doctor, nurse, and upperclassman to precede us in line for the elevator and through doors (not by choice, but as instructed). And anytime a doctor came into our presence on the halls we were expected to stand unless he gave permission to sit. We certainly were reminded where we fit into this caste system. No wonder we loved the stretcher boys—they were our equals.

Another rule was that we couldn't have a car at school. Too Easy—for all the rest of us!

Amazingly, Johnie Johnson has a car—a new one at that—and she brings it to school. She just parked it on side streets. She had a lot more luck hiding that than we did the cats and dogs in the dorm. She rarely drove the car in Temple—certainly not to classes. We did go for drives out of town sometimes, and to clubs or movies at night. Even the car couldn't make her into an ordinary chick though. We still didn't understand her.

October 18th was the first time for some of the girls to go on the halls to work. My turn wasn't for a couple more days. We started with one patient—giving morning care. Mine was a Mrs. Burton. She was rather obese and dipped snuff. I was scared stiff and seemed to get tangled in the curtains surrounding the bed while attempting to give her a bath.

Maybe they didn't know how much recreation some of us were having—or they just let us join the good girls who deserved a break—but there always seemed to be something planned for us by the school or the nurses association. We were feted with a big Halloween party—complete with bobbing for apples, a movie, and refreshments.

We became attached to a girl from Mexico, whose parents were going through the clinic. Georgette spent as much time in the dorm as we did for a couple of weeks. Peggy, Dottie, Shirley, and I even took her to the Shangri-La. Others, like Jimmie Lou, Shirley Marks, and a boy named Rueben (from TJC), were such frequent guests that they almost seemed part of the class.

Everyone had about four days off for Thanksgiving, and all went home to visit our parents. Joyce Lott and I took the train together to Houston—split up for buses to Beaumont and Livingston--then met and came back together after Thanksgiving.

On November 30th Carol and I went to see the movie, *White Christmas*. We had student discount tickets at the Arcadia. All of us spent a lot of our free time (and money) there.

There is a little Catholic church a few blocks from the dorm. I had never been inside one before Joyce Lott started taking me along on her sojourns. We usually go during the afternoon when no one else is there. The door is never locked. We cover our heads, and Joyce has a rosary—I assume she says prayers. We sit in absolute silence. It's a mystical experience for me, and a palpable presence always seems to hover about our pew.

Many of us fell in love with a hairstyle called a "duck." Don Bodenheimer may not have invented it, but might as well have had the patent as far as we were concerned. His barbershop was conveniently located next to one of the classrooms. And he was conveniently affordable. He always told jokes while he cut our hair, but he talked in such a whispery voice that I never heard one of the punchlines, and didn't dare ask him to repeat. Maybe he was funny—and maybe he was something else!

Dissecting frogs left such a lingering odor on our hands that some of the class had trouble eating meat after anatomy class. Dottie found that passing her hand under the nose of certain impressionable individuals could result in having their portion suddenly transferred to her plate.

Everyone had the Christmas spirit by the first of December. The dorm was decorated and looked great. On December 13th we had a class Christmas party and exchanged gifts. I had Dottie's name. The whole class went out caroling later. On December 14th the Junior class came to our dorm and sang carols for us. On December 16th the hospital had a Christmas party for the entire staff. It was held in the cafeteria and had a railroad theme. Tables were done up to look like cars from a train, and they were loaded with all types of goodies—the kind you see in your dreams.

The school had a tradition of giving a formal Christmas dance for the students. This year it was in the Hawn Hotel. It was one of those nice little things with all the faculty attending, and even some of the doctors. It was a chance to show what ladies we were. All the upperclassmen seemed to have dates and were appearing in their finery. Most of our motley crew couldn't come up with escorts. Some attended in a group. Margie had a date, and for some reason, had her mother's car. Dottie, Peg, and I ended up with the car. We dressed in our formal gowns (mine was borrowed from Darnell Thompson) and started for the party. We were inspired to improvise as we saw three young men in uniform walking downtown. They were delighted to join us. It was apparent from the look on Miss Cole's and Miss Gallman's faces that we hadn't fooled anyone. The trip through the assembly line was a disaster—as we were expected to introduce our escorts (we had neglected to ask their names). There was never another Christmas dance—not while we were in school!

The much anticipated trip home for the holidays finally arrived. Some of us had to wait until after Christmas day for our turn— since we were divided into two shifts.

Dottie decided that the holidays called for a special celebration. Eggnog was just the ticket! None of us had ever had eggnog, much less made it. Dottie came up with a bottle of bourbon (courtesy of Mr. Stroud), and smuggled it into the dorm. Carol, Lou, Peggy, Dottie, Joyce Lott, Shirley, and I barricaded ourselves in my room and proceeded to make some kind of drink out of eggs, milk, pecans, and bourbon. It was quite foul We had to hold our noses and force it down, but we swallowed enough to become rather inebriated. Lou, Carol, Joyce, and I had to be on duty on Hall II at seven the next morning. Everyone managed to keep their dry heaves to a minimum except Carol. She spent most of the morning at the water fountain—giggling. Lou and I kept reminding her not to drink so much water. We had some idea that it would make us drunk again. In Carol's case, it did! Stella May didn't say a word to us. She either didn't suspect the roots of our strange behavior, or chose to let it go.

Several people were assigned to remove the Christmas decorations and store them away. Time passed, and the dorm remained in the spirit of the holidays. The girls responsible were campused. In a rare fit of rebellion, Joni walked out of the dorm and took a long stroll around the neighborhood to prove that she had been wronged.

January 24th was the beginning of our pharmacology course. We love Mr. (Dr.) Jeffers. He enjoys answering questions and even lets us hang out in the pharmacy sometimes.

We also started doing procedures on patients. Maybe that was the impetus for our practical jokes since we were all a little giddy from the pressure of performing. Every day there was some new atrocity in the dorm as we tried to top each other. Cellophane would appear under the toilet seat during the night to catch the first one up. Light bulbs were unscrewed and cold cream applied. Beds were short sheeted every time someone was out. A few awful people even went so far as to sew up the legs and arms on other people's favorite pajamas. Drawers were exchanged in dressers—so that when you opened your drawer to get dressed—nothing was familiar. One group drank the tequila out of Joyce Helbert's souvenir bottle in her dresser drawer and filled the bottle with water. Eventually it got so out of hand that tempers started to flare and the pranks stopped.

Sharing clothes became another bone of contention. The problem was that some people borrowed clothes without permission. You might think you saw yourself going out on a date—and it was only your dress! The very worst was when you had slaved to iron something and didn't get to wear it first. (Of course, I think Peggy was the only one foolhardy enough to iron dozens of outfits at a time and leave them so temptingly available in her closet.) Jewelry (specially earrings) made the rounds also—as did things like Frenchie's lovely detachable collars.

Big skirts were the style. But the ruffled petticoats were what made them great. A few owned crinolines, but the rest of us made ours from yards and yards of muslin and saturated them with starch. I don't know how we sat down!

We suspected that the school really owned us, but we found how thoroughly when Dottie decided to pierce Lou's ears in the dorm. She carefully covered the bloody strings with clip-on earrings for the first excursion to the dining hall. Maybe it was those x-ray eyes, but it only took a short time for Miss Krempin to call Lou in and tell her that the strings would be removed forthwith.

We discovered Belton Lake. It became one of our prime spots for sunbathing. The moonlight wasn't bad either—quite often our dates ended up there on week-ends.

Riverside Pool in Belton was also a popular place—despite the gut wrenching smell of a rendering plant that we were obliged to drive past. We went in groups when we could get a car. Few of us could really swim—we waded in the shallow end—Ruthie making the biggest spectacle of herself, as she refused to wear her glasses in the pool and had to be led around.

An anonymous donor sent over a television set for our dorm. The sitting room became very popular as we vied for seats to watch our favorite programs. We couldn't miss Tennessee Ernie Ford and sometimes made the bus wait while we caught the last few minutes. A sitcom called *The People's Choice* was on in the evenings. It featured a dog that we all loved--a basset hound as I recall. A couple of weekly variety shows—the *Martha Raye Show*, and the *Show of Shows* with Sid Caesar and Imogene Coco—also kept us entertained.

Joyce Helbert had a date that didn't show up but called an hour later to apologize and tell her he had been in an accident. She found the next day that he had died shortly after the call. Only Joyce would have a date with such manners.

Someone discovered that we could purchase a sewing machine by paying monthly installments. It was the only thing we ever all agreed on, or owned jointly. Even the "non-seamstress" babes faithfully paid their share.

By April we were working seriously on the halls. It was still only about three hours a day, but with a bit more variety in duties. I was at 4&5 Cottages. We only learned to love Mary Belle Brown later when she worked in the West Building. Maybe it was the cottages (which were sometimes referred to as the cabbage patch) that turned her into a harridan. Most of our time in the cottages was spent giving endless enemas and douches. When we weren't actively pursuing some orifice, we were washing and boiling the tubes and cans. Dottie found how important it was to complete the cleaning process once after she received a call in the dorm from Mrs. Brown to return to the unit to remove her enema tubes from solution. The punishment was doubled by the embarrassment of a public reprimand and having to go through the process of dressing in her uniform again to make the trip over.

We giggled in the dorm as we recounted our problems and errors. I doubt that Miss Bohls, Miss Gallman, or Miss Cole were as amused. Our favorite story that came out of the first attempts at patient care was from Johnie Johnson. She had carefully bathed her patient, then decided to finish the job with a few sprays of under-arm deodorant. It turned out to be a sticky, yellowish, prescription nasal spray.

On April 26th we had our most traumatic anatomy lab. Dr. Daniels had us catch a stray cat that was hanging around the drug store. He proceeded to confine it in a large container and have some of the more hardy souls in the group give it drop ether. When the cat started screaming, at least half of us mutinied and ran out on the sidewalk. It became a rather interesting procedure after the cat was asleep. We all returned and watched the good doctor cut into the chest—crowding closely to watch the heart beating and the lungs expanding. We knew from the beginning that there would be no recovery and long convalescence for the cat. It didn't have much of a funeral either.

Cats didn't have a lot of luck around us. We either adopted one—or it adopted us. We hadn't had it in the dormitory long when we heard from Miss Cole—telling us that we would have the cat out immediately or she would personally come over and take care of it. We could just see her wringing its scrawny little neck, so we borrowed a car and drove the hapless kitty to Bruceville-Eddy and dropped it off in the middle of town. Then cried all the way home.

Johnie Johnson finally decided that some cowboy that worked at the Royal Club was more interesting than school. She departed with hardly a good-bye. I'm really going to miss her clothes.

Drugs and Solutions. It may be only another form of math, but it seems like six weeks of torture to me. I'm only surviving because Wanda Jo tutors me every day. I see X's in my sleep!

Dottie was the first of our class to be admitted to the hospital. She went in on May 22nd. There was a special room on North End for ailing students. But, you had to be <u>really</u> ill to be admitted, and being in the hospital was the only way to miss a day of work or class.

We found that Joyce Lott wasn't coming back after the class break. It was a blow to all of us.

On May 26th, after a day of anticipation and excitement, we went through the capping ceremony at 7:30 P.M. It felt good! Walking down the church aisle with our lighted Nightingale Lamps added to the drama of the night.

We all had a three week vacation. It was to be our only break for the summer. A time to visit with our families and catch them up on our progress. I, for one, regaled mine with the most gory details of hospital procedures and happenings.

On June 16th we were back at Scott and White. Along with the privilege of wearing our caps came more responsibility. We started immediately on eight hour shifts, except for class days, when our class hours were worked into that—giving us clinical hours of either 6-10 A.M., 7-11 A.M., or 4-8 P.M. We're now in Psychology and Medical Nursing.

Wanda Jo also chose marriage, and departed from our midst. She was a class favorite. Everyone will miss her very much.

Jane (name changed) started wearing a back brace, at first we believed the slipped disc thing, then we noticed a few changes in the front too. Even as naive as we were, we knew that back problems rarely caused the signs and symptoms she had begun to exhibit. We did talk about it among ourselves, but didn't tell anyone outside of the class—so obviously it was Jane who talked to Miss Cole. We knew we were in trouble when we were notified that Miss Cole would see the entire class (excepting Jane) in her office at one p.m. on July 19th. We were seated around a large conference table with Miss Cole at one end. She took off her glasses and shook them a few times, blue icicles shooting from her eyes. She asked each of us in turn what we had said about Jane. We were not allowed to give an easy answer. After an interminable time of pouring humiliation and guilt on us, she said, "this rumor is causing harm to an innocent girl, and has no basis in fact. This hospital can do without all of you very well, and if I hear another word about this, you will all find yourselves packing."   We filed out—a mass of human misery—specially Dottie, since Miss Cole singled her out to suggest a bit more time on her knees in church. I don't think any of us even dared let a stray thought enter our heads about Jane from that moment on. I, for one, averted my eyes when she walked around the dorm without the brace.

We were given physical exams again on July 20th.

On July 28th we had a watermelon party at Fifth Street Dorm. Peggy won the watermelon eating contest. Perhaps Jane should have!

It's quite warm in the dormitory, and we're always thirsty. The ice machine on North End does double duty to keep up with our forays across the street. The close proximity of a linen closet makes it easy to grab a pillow case to fill with the tempting cubes.

A big trauma at work for the several of us working on II West! We had become very attached to a patient named Mr. Brite. After a long hospital stay, he and his wife were packing up to go home on August 9th, and he suddenly died. We all worked the rest of our shift in only slightly controlled hysteria.

Celebrated my 20th birthday on the 18th of August. It turned out to be a big day! Carol gave me $1.50 (God knows where she got it!) Dot gave me a box of stationery. Shirley (Bob) gave me a pair of black bikini panties that I doubt I ever wore—I did prize them highly though. Just knowing they were there in the drawer added a bit of spice to my life.

September 1st. The new pre-clinical class moved in. It's an army! Twenty-four bright shining faces. At last, we're "upperclassmen."

They lied to us though! No one waits for us at the elevator. It's funny how rules change when it gets to be your turn.

One of our favorite pastimes was walking downtown—or just walking around in groups. We always had something to talk and giggle over. On a memorable trip, Peggy, Carol, Dottie, Lou, and I tried to lose some soldiers who had followed us—Carol finally resorted to pretending to have an epileptic seizure. (Perfect for our humanitarian image--mimicking the disabled—but Carol's performance was an award winner.)

Dot and I partied, then slept at the Strouds' home in Belton on Saturday night, September 24th. We spent the day Sunday blissfully unaware of the drama unfolding in the dormitory. Jackie and Sue had been dismissed from the school by Miss Cole. They stayed out without permission the night before. Jackie didn't plan to return—she had already made a decision to leave, but she neglected to let Sue in on the secret. Sue, ever easy to convince after a few drinks, agreed to spend the night out with Jackie and friends. Someone did confide in Miss Cole though. As soon as Sue stepped into the dorm on Sunday, there was a phone call telling her that she had an hour to pack and move out. No discussion!

We started a foods class in October at Temple Junior College. It was fun for most of us, but Lou cried every time her efforts failed.

We did get to eat what we cooked, and we never turned it down—
even Lou managed to swallow a few bites through her tears.

Dr. Harold Wood had become a particular favorite with the entire
class. He and his wife lived in the married interns housing across
from our dormitory. "Woody" was a good listener and had the
knack of making us feel that he was really interested in our lives.
We spent a lot of our free time hanging around and soaking up his
charisma. Of course, at the time, it wouldn't have raised many eye-
brows (except Miss Cole's), but he frequently gave us unwanted
bottles of prescription medicine samples that he received in the
mail. (This was when pharmaceutical companies sent out samples
by the hundreds to any intern or resident they could find.) He had
no idea that we would ever be stupid enough to take any of the
pills, but "some" of us were. What a great lawsuit that would have
made in later years!

I guess we hadn't had the class on fainting yet--the night that Lou
passed out cold at the Shangri-La. Carol, Peggy, Frenchie, and I
could only think to take her to the emergency room—sure that she
was dying. The actual emergency room was closed at night.
Woody was on call, and he met us in whatever room was used after
hours. Woody told us that he didn't need our help to examine her
but succumbed to our insistence. The four of us stood around the
examining table--providing only a lot of unprofessional giggling
(possibly a result of beer consumed earlier). Keeping his cool, under less than desirable circumstances, Dr. Wood pronounced her
well and sent us home to bed.

Someone in the dorm had a phonograph that played only "45's."
We were all in love with rock and roll" and "rhythm and blues."

Even in our impoverished state the newest hits often appeared, and everyone gathered around like moths to a flame. Dottie never tired of being the dance instructor, but even she couldn't turn the rest of us into Ginger Rogers.

We did like other music. Andy allowed us to play her albums once in a while. We wore new grooves into the Student Prince drinking song. And we even listened when Frenchie played classics on the piano.

Several of the class became serious smokers. I doubt that any of us had ever had a cigarette before nursing school. Smoking in uniform was strictly forbidden, so the smokers learned to take off their caps and shoes as soon as they returned to the dorm (making them officially out of uniform).

The nurses association gave us another Halloween party. Several of us dressed in costume.

On October 28th, Carol, Peggy, Frenchie, Dot, and I spent the day at Mr. and Mrs. Stroud's in Belton. Someone came up with the bright idea of making fudge. (I'm reasonably sure it wasn't Mrs. Stroud!) We walked around over town later, then snake danced along the streets.

Our screened in porch is always filled with dripping laundry. No washing machines for us! We wash everything in the lavatory. There is a Laundromat in the neighborhood, but where would we get the money? Luckily the hospital laundry keeps us supplied with clean starched and ironed uniforms. We're responsible for our own caps. Many a tear has been shed over scorching a cap and having to start over. I think Dottie would have sold her soul to anyone who would do the cap for her.

It snowed on November 8th. A group from our class trudged through the cold to 5th Street dorm tonight to help some of the pre-clinicals with their homework.

We all passed Medical Nursing. Started Surgical Nursing on November 9th.

The chore of guest lecturer fell to doctors doing their residency in that field at the time. Dr. Barrow left a lasting impression. I don't think any of us ever fell asleep in his class—we were mesmerized by him. The greenish shadows under his eyes added interest to an otherwise Montgomery Clift'ish face, and his voice was a throaty baritone. He chain smoked through every lecture and "French inhaled." The smoke, mingled with a decidedly sexual aura, encircled his head like a wreath.

We were having a lot of student association meetings. I don't know what we learned from them. Also the group parties continue. Mrs. Shehorn hosted one at her home.

By December Suzy was back in Temple working at Smitty's Restaurant. She frequently visited in the dorm but had an apartment with another waitress.

We were moved into Junior Dormitory while ours underwent a much needed renovation. That dorm never felt like home. We managed to give it our own brand of magic though. After a really fun night at the Shangri-La, we brought Carol back to the dorm in a state of inebriation. I was scheduled to work 11-7, and my date was waiting to walk me over. While I was getting into my uniform, Carol decided to stroll into the sitting room to talk to Tom— apparently forgetting that we had dressed her in a little strapless green teddy. Lou and I determined the thing to do was tie her in bed with scarves and belts so that she wouldn't wander off after we went to work. It happened to be my bed we chose. When I came in to go to sleep the next morning there was no Carol around. I blissfully slept several hours—then noticed a smell when I woke up. On moving my pillow it was obvious that "someone" had thrown up on it and just turned it over. Well, at least Carol didn't aspirate and die. Try explaining that one to Miss Cole!

Lou and I did return demonstrations on each other with our first intravenous stick. We were only injecting harmless vitamin C into the vein, but we both broke out in a cold sweat and held our breath as we watched the other closely to see that no air bolus was injected along with the solution. Unfortunately, we were both infatuated with the same boy at the time and were blessed with rather vivid imaginations.

Carol met Ed Ball at the Shangri-La. For some reason she was mortified when we played the "Eddie My Love" record at earsplitting level just as he picked her up for a date.

Had a Christmas tree and party in the dorm on December 13th. Apparently the food left something to be desired since we all rushed to the dining hall to eat as soon as it was over. The student association party was the next night. On the 15th our group party was held at Mrs. May's home, where we were served sandwiches and hot chocolate, then talked and watched television.

Marjorie got married over the holidays, but will remain in school. Maybe now Curtis will settle down. I guess our job is over. And just as we were getting good at fielding Curtis's constant phone calls and surveillance of the dorm—in search of his sometimes elusive love. (Of course, we didn't do too well the day he came into the dorm in a jealous rage and bounded up the stairs to find her—not a soul volunteered to tackle him.)

A bit of excitement on January 19th—a group of boys (showing off for their dates) misjudged the distance from the fire hydrant as they drove on our front lawn. The decapitated main looked like "Old Faithful" until the fire department arrived.

We started Public Health Nursing on January 23rd. A trip to the local sewerage plant grossed us all out, but the meat packing plant was even worse. We were all happily eating the free hot dog they gave us during the lovely tour through the sterile looking plant, when suddenly we found ourselves in a large room where a cow came through a chute and was hit in the head with a sledge hammer. We all exited the door so fast that we almost knocked each other down. The half eaten hot dogs went into the trash bin. (I think that part of the process could have been left to our imagination.)

The entire student body worked together to prepare an area for a volleyball court behind Fifth Street dorm. We raked, shoveled, and moved rocks—then someone came in and poured concrete. I think our class used it very little after it was completed, other than the group party held on January 26th—with volleyball games and a hot dog roast.

We all went to church on Sundays—sometimes at night during the week also. On February 1st Miss Andy, Ruthie, Sammie, Lou, Joyce, and I attended prayer service together on a Wednesday night, and went to Smitty's for a coke after.

Our group party for February was on the 16th at Mrs. Pargin's. She served us popcorn—and another round of television.

Fourteen student nurses were "honor guards" at Dr. Scott's funeral on February 23rd. (I wasn't even a guest.)

Dr. Linss was our surgical nursing lecturer until March 1st, when Dr. Rodriquez took over. The class watched a tracheotomy tube changed on Four West on March 6th.

I was back working at 4&5 Cottages in March. Our early morning duties usually included preparing patients to go for surgery. Lou and I both gave narcotic pre-op's to the wrong patients during this tour. Of course, Lou and I seemed to follow each other into trouble often. Dr. Birdwell was sitting at the nurses station when I reported my error in medication. Never one to pass up a chance—he said, "quick, run and draw it back out". He routinely wrote tongue in cheek orders on patient charts, like the one for an elderly farmer, "scrub feet with kerosene and a corn cob." One of his post-op orders on another patient was, " may commune with nature at will." Many of our patients in the cottages were sent to the main building and the clinic for surgery and diagnostic procedures. It was the duty of the ever present "stretcher boys" to transport them on the bumpy ride across a fairly busy street. There was no covered walkway, and on rainy days covers were fashioned from tarpaulin. If a student was elected to accompany the patient—an umbrella was sometimes available—and sometimes she just got wet!

Does anyone know what stupes really do? And has anyone ever done them without getting the scalding water on their own hands? I wonder about many tailed binders too. What are they holding in— and does it fall out if they aren't applied correctly?

On March 8th our class gave two performances of a skit called, "Princess for an Hour" —once for the alumni association and then for the district nurses meeting.

Jerry (last name omitted) lost his temper at the Shangri-La and got in a terrible fist fight with a guy named Nickie. (Something about who was going to dance with Dottie.) It seemed to go on for ages—all over the dance floor—with blood flying and the sickening sound of knuckles hitting flesh. We all left, so I don't know if the police were called. The owners closed the Shangri-La from that date (March 10th) to April 6th. The sign said that it was closed for repairs, but it might as well have been closed for good. It was never the same again. We did hang out there, but the huge crowds just never came back.

On March 15th the group party was at Mrs. Brown's home.

Even Sam went out to the movies once in a while. On March 23rd she, Lou, Joni, and I went to the Arcadia.

Lou, Ruthie, Carol, Frenchie, Joyce, and I started in surgery to- gether on March 26th. It was intimidating—to say the least. We all felt very dumb. Of course, we weren't allowed to hand instruments to the surgeons. They all had their own nurses. Mostly we scrubbed in and observed. We did do an awful lot of instrument and glove washing. I guess they thought we were qualified for that. (All the gloves were washed, checked for holes, and re-sterilized. What a job!) Actually, I think we only rotated through the instrument room for a week. It just seemed like longer. Dr. Brindley Sr. probably gave us the most vivid memories to take away. He always threw his hat as he strolled into the hallway in the mornings. A student was expected to catch it and hang it on the hall tree. He also taught us the meaning of "pour girl pour." Lou had one special reason to remember him. As she was observing a mastectomy (unscrubbed) one day, he said, "Girl, take this to the lab." She hesitated too long in her quandary about the necessity for sterile technique. He lobbed a large breast at her chest, and it slid down to the floor. Sometimes we were allowed to close a case with the surgical residents. Dr.'s Linss and Hayden let me pass sutures to them several times. We six students had to scrub in one day and remove all the flesh from an amputated leg—after watching the surgical procedure. (The bones were saved for the bone bank.) We managed to get through it without throwing up! They probably served us some more saltines and milk after we finished. (I couldn't eat saltine crackers for years after my stint in surgery.) We were assigned to be on call, but since we had no responsibility in surgery, it had to be for the experience of getting up in the middle of the night. I was only called in once. Seven patients involved in an auto accident were admitted for surgery. Most of the injuries were fractures and lacerations. When I was awakened from a sound sleep at 11:30 at night I was disoriented and panic stricken. I threw on my clothes and rushed over (sure that I would be sole care giver for all those people). When I arrived in surgery, I realized that I didn't have on a bra under my scrub dress. I spent most of the time trying to keep my arms folded across my chest. That's tough to do while taking blood pressure readings—which, of course, turned out to be my only assignment.

Lou kept wearing her worn out nursing shoes in surgery because her mother had promised to buy her new ones (and Lou certainly wasn't going to spend her stipend money on that if she could help it). They must have been pathetic because one of the nurse anesthetists called her aside one day and gave her money to buy a new pair. She was embarrassed, but certainly not enough to turn the money down!

Muriel had a laminectomy while we were on surgery rotation. Our group was allowed to watch the procedure. It was strange, and rather unsettling, to watch doctors cut into one of our own.

They had us work in x-ray to observe arteriograms while we were on surgery rotation. Also went along to Santa Fe hospital for some surgeries. I was scrubbed in on a thyroidectomy one day, and the surgeon had me break scrub and go in the other room to lie down. He thought I was going to faint, and didn't want me on his sterile field. I was humiliated that he thought I couldn't stand the sight of blood. It had nothing to do with the surgery—just "death" by menstrual cramps.

We did learn a lot about sterile technique in surgery. And all those close up encounters with anatomy couldn't have been found in a book.

On April 10th "Jane" visited the dorm. I can't imagine how she had the nerve.

Dr. Happock is one of our guest lecturers in class. He talked about feet on the 12th.

What was with all the singing? Were we trying out for something? We seemed to sing everywhere we went. On April 18th after a spaghetti dinner that we cooked in the popcorn popper, we sang in the dorm, then went to Betty Wood's and serenaded her for a couple of hours. (No wonder we ate first—those vegetarian hot-dogs she served were pretty bad. Betty didn't eat meat for religious reasons.) Muriel was still in the hospital on April 21st. I spent three hours with her. I think we sort of alternated doing special duty.

The seniors are returning from affiliation.

Ramon Carreno fell for Lou while she was working in surgery. He had her hold his expensive watch and ring while he scrubbed every day. Sometimes she forgot to give them back, and the jewelry spent the night in the dorm. Once I kept them in my room for safe keeping while Lou went out on a date (with someone other than Ramon).

Lou and I went on a double date with Dr. Carreno and Dr. Aguilar. We drove to Waco to have dinner and went to a movie. They were fun and easy to be with. Unfortunately, the next time they invited us out, it was to go to the Stagecoach Inn for dinner. We built up our anxiety about how to dress to a point that we foolishly decided that a "harmless" Thorazine would be just the thing to smooth us out for the evening. (Our pills came from Woody's gifts). Dinner was fine, but by the time we were dancing at the S&S my pill had kicked in (aided by a couple of drinks). After almost falling on Carlos, I confided what we had done. We were lectured on our mental state, and immediately returned to the dorm. We sure impressed them!

Can anyone forget the interminable time we spent one night in Classroom II watching slides of Dr. Valiente Gracia's vacation in Mexico?

Or his trying to get us into closets at work?

Dottie and I were assisting with a spinal tap in a treatment room, and she fainted dead away—hitting the floor with a thud, and knocking over equipment in the process. (It was a very small room.) It was probably one of her most embarrassing moments. The doctor and I were so rattled we couldn't decide whether to take time to reassure the patient first or to check on Dottie.

Betty Wood moved back to Memphis on April 27th. We had an ice cream party for her. Woody is staying on to finish his internship.

We were always hungry—despite the fact that we were fed three large meals a day. The food in the cafeteria was actually rather good, but we were constantly looking for something to supplement our diet. Besides cooking in the popcorn popper, we ate at Veteran's Cafe, Smitty's, Janeway's Drug, or the Shangri-La whenever we could find the extra money. Snappy's Drive Inn was another favorite. We found that a cab would deliver our order of hamburgers after curfew. I'm sure the driver loved our 10 cent tips.

The diner next to our dormitory also made sandwiches. We mostly bought cokes and doughnuts from them though. They were nice to us because we were students and didn't charge us the deposit on our

coke bottles (depending on us to return them). As it turned out—
some of us were taking the bottles to a grocery store for a refund—
it was great movie money. It was a little embarrassing when the
owners of the diner reminded us that they knew the bottles weren't
coming back.

On May 9th Woody took almost the entire class for a picnic at Riverside. We all crowded into his car for the trip. It was very cozy.

Woody decided that a puppy would be a great gift for us. We
smuggled it into the dorm and named it "Woo." Woo lasted only
long enough to eat all of our shoes and sweaters before Miss Cole
got wind of him. I don't recall what we did with him, I just know
that he was out in a hurry. I'm pretty sure that Woody took him
back.

We were treated to another sunrise breakfast at 5:30 a.m. on May
12th. We still had enough energy left over to play a softball game
with the interns and residents on our lawn later.

I don't know how we ever played games—or even walked on that
lawn—it was solid grass burrs. The little circle of bluebonnets was
pretty in the Spring, but the rest of the year the burrs were the
prominent feature.

Had my second hospital admission on May 29th. Dottie and I went
to Belton Dam with dates the night before. We were supposedly
having a going away party for Dot's current boyfriend. We sat in
the dark on a bluff overlooking the lake and drank gin and grapefruit juice. Dot kept letting them refill her glass—so I did also.
Since Dottie didn't even drink—I was sure that they weren't very

strong. As it turned out—Dottie was pouring her drinks in the dirt.
My date (whom I never saw before or after) obviously wasn't pouring his drinks out. It was his car, and he kept saying he was going
to drive off a cliff on the way home. I was sort of hoping he would.
I was lying in the back seat with my head in Dottie's lap—just trying to breathe without throwing up. When I pried myself out of
bed the next morning to go to work I thought I was dying. I took
another of Woody's trusty Thorazines. I made it to II West, but
during report I had to keep getting up and having dry heaves over
the sink. I must have looked awful because the charge nurse took
me in an empty room and gave me an injection of Thorazine. She
said, "I'll kill you if you ever tell". I didn't have the nerve to tell her
that I had already taken 25 mgm. When I didn't improve, Mrs.
Brown sent me to the dorm to lie down. She became worried when
I didn't return in an hour, and sent Carol to check on me. I couldn't
stand up—so they transported me to the hospital in a wheel chair.
Of course, I couldn't tell Dr. Hammond that I had taken either
Thorazine. I assured him that I had eaten something that made me
ill. He gave me a Nembutal, and admitted me to the hospital. I
slept for about 48 hours. When I sneaked a look at my clinic chart
later, I saw that he had written for a diagnosis, "gastritis?" Hard to
fool that man!

On June 4th Ruthie was excused to go home for her grandfather's
funeral.

Muriel was recovered enough to go swimming at Belton Lake on
June 4th with Dot, Sam, and me—and four guys.

Muriel met Ron Clarke, and they were married after dating for a
short while. They moved into an apartment near the dorm. It was a

great place to sleep when we needed overnight permission to stay out past curfew.

Woody loaned us his car several times after Betty left. Usually we used it to drive to Belton Lake to swim. Frenchie and I did take the car to the Cascade one night also.

Woody's internship was completed and he was getting ready to join Betty in Memphis by the second week of June. He and Dr. Pat McGowan went out to the Shangri-La and got quite drunk to celebrate on the night of the 14th . (Even we were embarrassed by them.) Carol and I helped Woody pack the car the next day. He left with every inch of the car filled with boxes and clothes— leaving only enough room to sit to drive. It must have been near impossible to see where he was going. I do believe that he had the dog (Woo) with him also.

The clinical part of Foods and Nutrition class began at Santa Fe on June 18th. The instructor allowed us to watch Tennessee Ernie Ford on television every day before we started class. Most of the class time was spent writing special diets. Joyce had the use of her mother's car (and permission to drive us), so we had a chauffeur. Her parents lived near the hospital, and sometimes we walked over after class to get the car—having to trudge through a gully on the short cut. This stint was a fun time—with no pressure. (Joyce's constant singing of all the verses of "Que Sera" did jangle a few nerves.) We spent a lot of time looking at the goldfish in the pond by the hospital—and diagnosing them with cancerous tumors. Our skills became a bit suspect when we found later the "tumors" were actually wounds from vandals.

I started O. B. rotation on July 16th. Scrubbed in and watched my first delivery. It was a girl. She was named Rita Margaret Pinkham.

Dot, Carol, and I were on O. B. call to Cora Anderson and went over to watch a birth at 10:30 P. M. We stayed around until 1:30 in the morning. That hospital held an aura of mystery for us. We hardly ever actually worked there.

Had physicals again on the 20th of July. I think we all passed!

Carol went home to Shamrock for her summer vacation. She came back as Mrs. Ed Ball.

NBC Matinee Theater became one of our new favorites on television.

Since Lou, Frenchie, and I had birthdays near each other—we decided to bake a cake. Mary Belle Brown allowed us to use her kitchen. I don't recall how good the cake was, but I do remember that it was chocolate, and it fell apart. We had to splice it together with tooth picks.

Either we had been extra good—or Andy was tired of the routine of cafeteria food too. On August 20th, she treated us to "carry out" chicken, and we had dinner in the dorm.

Had a group party at Mrs. Tune's house and spent the time playing our favorite card game, "I Doubt It."

I went home for three week summer vacation. Spent several days with a cousin in Beaumont—so I had the opportunity to visit Joyce Lott at her new nursing school. (A bit disappointed that she was getting along great without us!)

Came back to the dorm to find Suzy had been re-admitted to nursing school. Her father talked Miss Cole into giving her another chance. She'll be a year behind us, but it's exciting to have her back.

Elvis Presley made his debut on the Ed Sullivan Show. I was working 3-11, but a patient invited me to watch it on a television in his room. I didn't dare take time out for the entire performance, but did catch passing glimpses.

Started in Public Health on September 17th. Mrs. Wilson and Mrs. Bond took us on home visits.

Carol and Ed were in a car accident on September 23rd. Luckily no one was injured.

Whether we did it as a favor to Dr. Hightower, to help with his research project, or for the five dollars they paid us, we were pretty stupid to agree to be guinea pigs. We four "volunteers" were given a medication to take daily for a week (mine was Probanthine). At the end of the week we had to swallow a gastric tube with a balloon on the end, and lie on a hard x-ray table for about four hours with the inflated balloon holding the tube in place. Dr. Hightower and an assistant aspirated gastric contents for analysis and did some type of radiological imaging. I went through four boxes of Kleenex as I drooled around the tube. We were instructed to remain NPO after midnight before the procedure. I don't know about anyone

else, but I didn't exactly follow orders. I worked 11-7, the Probanthine made me terribly thirsty, and I spent most of the night drinking grapefruit juice from the unit kitchen. The only thing the doctors gleaned from my test was that my stomach was totally devoid
of acid. They told me that it probably meant I was prone to stomach cancer (either they flunked psychology, or suspected my trans-
gression and were punishing me).

Ruthie and I were working on III Clinic in October. Several times
guys we were dating came up to visit us. I guess we thought we
could get away with it since we worked at night in an isolated area
with very little supervision. As luck would have it, a house super-
visor came by one night while two young men were lounging near
the nurses station. We pretended not to know who they were, and
she ushered them unceremoniously out the door.

Boiling pots of enema tubes aren't to be trifled with. I managed to
get a third degree burn—covering the entire back of my left hand,
including all my fingers. I rushed over to see Dr. Hammond—
thinking he would miraculously cure it. He did absolutely nothing!
His only advice was that bathing patients would help it heal. I sup-
pose he was right. I didn't lose my hand, even though it went
through several very gross stages before it looked normal again.
One night while dancing at the Shangri-La, a date was holding that
hand, and said, "could I ask you something?" "Do you use Ponds?"

III Clinic was never a busy unit. When Sam worked there at night
she couldn't stay awake so she set the little timer that we had for
boiling enema tubes. She would sleep until the ten minute timer
went off—check the patients—then set the timer again. All of us
were amazed that "sweet Sam" was the only one of us with the

nerve to plan a nap at work.

Went to Houston for the week-end on November 5th. I visited my sisters, but helped Carol and Ed look for an apartment also. Carol and I made the return trip to Temple together on the train.

Ruthie was dating Don Flewell, and he sometimes loaned her his car. Lou, Ruthie, and I took the car to Belton Lake and washed it with lake water on November 13th. We flirted with pneumonia, but the car looked good! Lou, Frenchie, Ruthie, and I took the car to Killeen, just to ride around, on the 15th.

Shirley had a baby boy on the 16th of November at 11:45 A.M. (She dropped out of school after her marriage to L. E. Hill.)

Joyce and I worked alone on II West 11-7 on the 20th of November. We only had one LVN to take vital signs. We were beginning to know the meaning of responsibility. It was a very busy floor. We loved the patients there. It was probably the best place to work in the hospital. Mrs. McClaugherty, one of our favorites, was the 3 -11 charge nurse.

Don Flewell bribed a stretcher boy to loan him his white coat one day while Ruthie and I were working on II West. We tried to ignore him as he busily swept one of the halls, but finally succumbed to hysteria. Thankfully, Miss Cole didn't decide to pick that time for a walk through.

We were getting ready to go to Houston for affiliation by the last week in November. Had several parties in preparation for our departure.

The school gave us money for the train trip to Houston, but some of us opted to go by car. Dot's parents drove Dot and me. They dropped us off at the dormitory. It was such a shock to see where we were going to be living that I think Dot and I both cried. God knows we hadn't been living in the lap of luxury in the dorm at Scott and White, but at least it was homey. We were the first ones to arrive at the Jeff Davis dorm, and it looked about as inviting as a prison cell. The rooms each had one single bed and a metal dresser. The windows were covered by metal venetian blinds. The floors were marble. There was one large bathroom down a hall. It had a row of showers, a long lavatory counter, and several toilet stalls. By the time some of the others arrived, we had decided that we couldn't sleep there that night. Lou, Frenchie, Sue, Ruthie, Dot, and I stayed at my sister's and slept on the floor. Sue was just visiting with us while we moved in. She had to go back to Temple, and either by coincidence or design, Lou's brother, Jimmy was available to drive her.

On November 26th, we toured the hospital for orientation. I stupidly wore new shoes. My feet were bleeding while we walked all the halls and up and down stairwells, and I didn't dare complain.

Carol and Ed, and Marjorie and Curtis are living in apartments nearby.

The entire class walked downtown on November 29th. We explored the town for a while. When a suggestion came up that we go to the Silver Spur, the class divided in half as usual. One half went back to the dorm, and the rest of us spent a couple of hours watching and listening to Lavelle White. It quickly became our new

"Shangri-La." The owner of the club (Jimmy Menudas) must have enjoyed having us. When our group went in without escorts, he always served us free cokes. We walked to the Silver Spur most of the time. It was a nice walk during the day, but after dark was another thing entirely. We had to go through a seedy, all-black area where the street was lined with noisy overflowing bars and night clubs, spilling groups of men in our path on the narrow sidewalk. After getting past that obstacle, there was a long stretch by a cemetery with few or no street lights. Never discouraged us! If you want to dance, you must pay the piper!

O. B. at Jeff Davis was mostly a nightmare. The labor and delivery rooms were filled with screaming women (funny, they didn't scream at S&W). Each room held several women, just separated by curtains. Usually the curtains weren't even drawn. There was no room for modesty. The first time one of us tried to drape a patient for a vaginal exam the resident asked what we thought we were doing. Pubic preps were the worst assignment. Most of the Hispanic women had forests of hair starting at their belly buttons. Some of them probably retained permanent scars from our razors--since we were always rushed—as heads crowned. Roaches often ran across a sterile pack, and you didn't dare close it and get another. The Chief Resident (Dr. Dampeer) treated us like we were idiots. But labor and delivery was a picnic compared to postpartum. There was never enough linen for the beds, nor for bathing the patients. We were actually told to use one end of a towel for washing and the other for drying. Also when sheets were scarce, we used the old top sheet for a bottom sheet on the "clean" bed (even sometimes for a different patient.) I never saw so much blood! Did we use gloves? Roaches were a major problem. It was nothing to see a roach floating in the water pitcher at a bedside. The nursery was a bit of a zoo also. If the bassinets didn't have every inch scrubbed with disinfectant every day they would be swarming the next morning with new baby roaches vying for space with the human babies. Other than battling vermin, most of our time in the nursery seemed to involve bathing and weighing slippery newborns. I don't remember what we used for bathing, but I do recall how difficult it was to get a grip on those vernix covered bodies, and how challenging to get the silver nitrate solution in their squinty little eyes.

On December 19th we had a Christmas party in the sitting room on our floor. Our Christmas tree was pathetic, bringing on bouts of tears as we valiantly tried to trim it (with no real ornaments). Had a party in O. B. the next night. L & D was decorated with a lot of Santa faces and snow—mainly fashioned of bits of cotton from maxi-pads.

Only had four days off to go home for Christmas.

Joyce and I were assigned to ante-partum clinic together. I think blood pressure readings were our specialty. But we loved listening to the fetal heart tones when the doctors let us take a turn.

On New Year's Eve night Peggy, Lou, and I went to the Melody Club with our dates. Our group contained the only white faces. My ex-roommate-Joyce Malkey(pre nursing school) and her husband owned the black nightclub and invited us to be their guests. Her parents were there also. We all sat at a large table by the bandstand. It was very loud and a lot of fun. The only strange thing that happened was seeing a black lady rearrange a knife in the top of her stocking while we were in the ladies room. Joyce's father had brought me a bottle of homemade wine. I had to be in the dorm at midnight, and inadvertently left the bottle of wine in the car. Lou and Peggy denied drinking it, but I knew better. I was mad for days.

Of course, I was already feeling put upon that I had to cut short the night—while they stayed out and celebrated.

Started working on pediatrics the first week of January. And we thought O. B. was bad! The day shift was awful, but at least we were only assigned "several" difficult patients, since the staffing was usually adequate. On evenings there was one RN, and she was lousy. She also left at 10:20 sharp every night—even if all the kids were dying. Her husband picked her up at that time, and she never kept him waiting. There was no RN at night. It was often just one of us and a Prairie View student—with some of the worst nurses aides ever hired. The unit held over 60 very ill children. The aides on my side always spent more time sleeping than working. They would pour out the formula if the babies didn't drink fast enough— then hide in the linen closet and use stacked linens on a shelf for a pillow.

The pediatric floor had every kind of patient imaginable. Perhaps the worst was the burn ward—with patients covered in third degree burns. Just changing the dressings or sheets was a real trauma for us and the kids. One girl had to be soaked in a tub of Phisohex and water to loosen her bandages. She screamed through the entire pro-cedure—and could be heard several floors away. No picnic either was the diarrhea ward, nor the vast assortment of surgical and medical plights.

And if we thought linens were scarce on obstetrics, try finding a

real diaper on pediatrics! It was a miracle the days that we had
them. Often we folded whatever we could find into a reasonable
facsimile.

Both my sisters lived in Houston at the time. Frenchie, Lou, Dot,
and I spent the night with my older sister fairly often in order to
have overnight permission. In one poorly planned visit Dottie and I
walked from J.D. to Faye's house (about five miles); they weren't
home, and we had to walk back.

We became friends with several of the Prairie View students. They
lived in another dorm (a white frame two story building that looked
like a converted barracks). Segregation was in full sway, and the
Jeff Davis students were not thrilled that we had the P.V. girls in
our dorm for visits.

Joni and Robert went dancing with a group of us on January 27th.

I borrowed money from the maid to take the train to Temple for a
visit (fare was $5.00). Spent the night with Muriel and Ron (but I
was there to see a boyfriend, of course).

We loved Ruth (the maid in the dorm at Jeff Davis). And the feeling was mutual. She always had a sympathetic ear for our troubles,
and enjoyed listening to our chatter. Sometimes doughnuts magi-
cally appeared for breakfast when one of us had worked ll-7 and
felt too tired to go to the dining room. And if she knew an inspec-
tion was coming up she would always warn us—even help straigh-
ten up if time was tight. She knew we loved R&B music, and she
brought some of her own records over. But affection didn't stop her
from berating us and saying that we deserved to have something

happen to us when we walked home from downtown at night. She also insisted it was our fault the interns and medical students stopped the elevator on our floor—since we ran around in our nightgowns—and less.

There was a stationary door on each floor that had to be opened for the elevator. It had a small window in it. Once we drew an elaborate frowning face to cover the window to greet the future doctors and keep them from looking out on our floor. It lasted less than a day. A message came from the housemother that we must take it down immediately.

We worked a lot of 11-7 while we were in pediatrics. It didn't get us out of class the next day. Sometimes we had two hours of class before we could go to bed. Just staying awake through the class was a major accomplishment--learning was incidental.

On February 22nd. Lou, Dot, Peg, Frenchie, and I went to Carol and Ed's apartment and cooked a "delicious" dinner.

We had a good reason for our constant hunger at Jeff Davis. The food was gross in the cafeteria. Breakfast was always the same— scrambled powdered eggs, lukewarm orange and tomato juice, greasy bacon, and toast that seemed to have been dipped in melted margarine. Lunch at least had a little more variety, but wasn't any better. Possibly fearing that we would starve to death and they would have to explain sending our emaciated bodies back, the hierarchy allowed us to have dinner in the dining room reserved for doctors and RNs (after they finished, of course). Food was served family style. The best part being the pitchers of iced tea and hot rolls and butter. We survived on those when nothing else was ap-

petizing. Often we had to resort to smothering the food with catsup—specially the mystery meat. When we worked 11-7 sandwiches were served in the dining room. We never had enough time
for a break—so didn't know if these were more palatable. As an
added inducement to eat—bread, eggs, butter, chocolate milk, and
regular milk were wheeled over from the dining room every
morning and placed in our refrigerator in the dorm. Strangely
enough, one of my most memorable sandwiches was made in the
Jeff Davis kitchen. They packed a lunch for us to take along when
we went out to spend the day in a child care center. Mine was a
thick slice of real roast turkey with lots of black pepper, lettuce, and
mayonnaise on white bread.

Marion Hunter and I took a city bus to the child care center. The
buses were still segregated of course, with blacks sitting in the
back. Marion and I sat in the front together. People stared, but did-
n't say anything. We looked so angelic in our uniforms and capes,
they probably didn't have the heart.

A "lovely" sitting room and kitchen were part of the living arrange-
ment on our floor in the dormitory. The sitting room had a sofa,
several chairs, a television, and a phone. We amused ourselves by
watching the mouse that lived in the sofa. (I once emptied him out
of the wastebasket in my room during the night—into a larger
wastebasket down the hall and went right back to sleep.) The view
from the window of the sitting room was straight into the parking
lot for the emergency room. The blaring of sirens became our
background music. Sammie was often seen staring out the window,
saying, "look at that parking lot". I don't know if she was amazed
or disgusted by the scenes unfolding below.

The kitchen was a cubicle holding a refrigerator, a small stove, and a dinette table with four chairs. The only time that I recall our cooking anything in the kitchen was the night that Peggy decided that she could make gravy without meat or drippings. It was concocted of flour, margarine, and milk. We ate it on bread with catsup. Delicious!!!! We did have a cake in the kitchen once. It must have been someone's birthday. During the night some of the Jeff Davis students crept up the stairs and stole the cake. They surely were very disappointed on their other forays onto our floor. We rarely had anything edible.

Now, drinkable was another thing! We smuggled beer (and once vodka) into the dorm, then dropped the empties down the laundry chute (they fell directly to the basement, so no one could prove which floor they originated on). (The "we" only included about five of us—the rest were teetotalers.) I signed in at the desk one night and was walking away from the housemother with a paper bag of beer—as I neared the elevator--the bag broke--beer cans went in several directions. I never looked back after I picked them up, just jumped into the elevator. She probably wasn't energetic enough to investigate the source of the clatter anyway.

The elevator in the dorm was the bane of our existence. Getting in it alone at night was an experience. It frequently went to the basement first—no matter what button was pushed. There was nothing scarier than the basement at night—except when the elevator decided to stop between floors—or go to the top where the medical students and interns lived.

Peggy's blood curdling scream woke us from a sound sleep sometime after midnight and several of us raced to her room—finding an intern trying to get in her bed and telling her to be quiet. His excuse later was that he thought he was on his floor and getting into his own bed. (Maybe he was used to someone already being in it.) The director of nurses bought it—or was too chicken to go against the doctors!

Joyce and I worked together a lot on pediatrics. We fell in love with several of the patients. They were difficult, hungry for affection, and, of course, very ill. One day I had to hold a boy to have his penicillin injection while Joyce gave it. He was almost as big as we were. He wouldn't lie down, so I had to wrap my arms around him—standing up—in a "lover's" embrace—while Joyce dropped his pajamas and injected him. He fought us and screamed bloody murder, but was all smiles after we finished. On February 28th we were working 3-11 when a four year old named Aurora Brown died. Joyce and I were in the treatment room with several medical students and interns. They insisted on inserting tubes and doing all kinds of tests on her—essentially desecrating her body for no obvious reason. It wasn't an autopsy! Joyce and I were quite distressed—didn't get back to the dorm until one in the morning—then couldn't sleep--so we sat and talked—and cried.

Note from one of my pediatric patients.

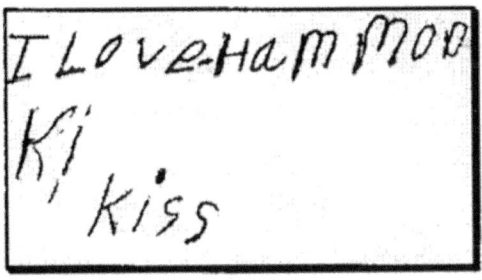

Made the mistake of telling the head nurse that I saw something crawling in a patient's hair. It turned out to be lice. Guess who had to do the treatment!!

An albino black girl in a body cast was mortally afraid of roaches, but they seemed to favor her. (Maybe it was the delightful aroma coming from under the cast.) She spent most of her time screaming, "ro-ach, ro-ach."

A three year old boy with a prolapsed rectum was a semi-permanent resident. I'm not sure anyone knew where his parents were. Dottie loved him—as did several other students. I couldn't stand to look at him. That errant part always seemed to be trailing out of his diaper.

We had an extensive case study to do in pediatrics. It counted for a major portion of our class grade. My sister, Faye, was an executive secretary. She took me to her office one night and typed mine on her electric typewriter. It was beautiful. I felt guilty about the A+ on the paper, even though I had done a tremendous amount of work on the content. I always suspected the instructors were blinded by the typing and formatting.

We all rotated through the outpatient clinic for pediatrics. It was a fun thing. The doctors and nurses in the clinic were great. We spent a lot of time talking to Dr. Milton. There was also a black doctor that we liked a lot. He loved talking and we sat in his office every time we had a break.

We also went out on rounds with a school nurse. I visited Braeburn Elementary. We checked for head lice. Lovely! I may never feel clean again.

Dot, Sam, and I discovered a cemetery across Buffalo Bayou from
the hospital. We spent several hours there one day. We had to
climb over the fence to get in. It was beautifully landscaped with
all kinds of plants. Wisteria, azaleas, roses, and numerous other
species were in bloom. There was a cat sleeping by one of the
mausoleums. We spent time on the grass with the cat, then explored the grounds. Very peaceful!

Premature nursery was a strange experience. The babies were like
toys. Some of them only weighed a pound or so. They looked like
little old men and women with wrinkled prune skin. We never held
the babies—just did nursing procedures through the arm holes in
the incubators. Feeding them was a real chore. Some could take a
bottle, but it seemed to take forever. Others were on IV's or were
fed through gastric feeding tubes.

On March 22nd, Dot, Lou, Frenchie, and I made one of our trips to
the Silver Spur—and Joyce went along (a really, really rare occur-
rence).

Ruth loaned us her car to look for boxes to pack our things. Ruthie,
Lou, Sam, Frenchie, and I drove around to area grocery stores.

We had boxes stacked around in the hallways for several days. I
have no idea what we planned to put in one very large box—since
our meager possessions would hardly warrant it. Lou convinced
me to get in the box, then recruited several others to hold the lid
down while they pulled the box into the elevator and pushed the
button. (I had just come from the shower, and my only attire was a

towel.) When I managed to get back to our floor—to kill Lou—she ran—hit the edge of a door—and broke her toe. We walked over to Pedi Clinic and had Dr. Milton look at the toe. He confirmed our diagnosis, but said only time would heal it. He couldn't do anything to speed it along. Lou limped for weeks.

Ruth gave us a going away party at her home on the 27th of March, and the entire class attended. She served drinks and food, but the most interesting thing was that every light bulb in her house was pink. We all looked great! She sent her husband and son to visit relatives. No men were allowed. It was just a girl thing.

While we were waiting in the dorm's main sitting room before going to Ruth's, Ed picked up a record and pretended to throw a discus. He accidentally lost his grip and threw it across the room—it shattered on a wall about ten feet away. Not a giggle nor a gasp out of the several Jeff Davis students in the room. They looked at us like we were visiting from another planet—and that was the kind of behavior they might expect.

That was an unfriendly group of nursing students. Maybe we did something to tick them off, but I don't believe one of them ever spoke to us.

Our instructors for pediatrics were Ann Smith and Ruth Shobert. They lived together—and were very good friends. As a going away gesture--they visited us on our floor in the dorm—bringing along their enormous German Shepherd dog.

Our last day at Jefferson Davis Hospital was March 31st. We left Houston at 10:30 a.m. and arrived in Galveston at 11:30. My sister drove Dot, Peg, and me to Galveston (my brother-in-law was along, but I'd prefer to edit him out). We spent the first afternoon on the beach. Had hamburgers and beer for dinner.

This dormitory bears no resemblance to our previous dwellings. We're in suites, consisting of two double occupancy rooms with a bathroom between. There is carpeting on the floor. The furniture is new and everything is *so* clean. We each have a desk with built in bookshelves above. The beds have great mattresses, and there is even a comfortable chair. The rooms look like a place someone would actually enjoy living. There is no housemother in sight. We were all given keys to the front door. What is this? A trick? Where is the real dormitory?

Carol and Marjorie were back in the dorm. (Curtis and Ed stayed in Houston.) Muriel and Shirley had returned to school, and were with us for affiliation. It was like old times.

We were assigned roommates alphabetically. Joyce and I are together. Frenchie with Lou. Dottie and Sam, Shirley and Ruthie, Marjorie and Peg, and Muriel with Carol.

Robert has moved to Galveston to join his bride, so Joni isn't in our dorm. They have an apartment in family housing across the street.

On April 1st we were up early, had breakfast at the cafeteria in family housing, and marched over to the hospital in a group—all dressed in our uniforms. Our class met the other affiliates, and all of us were oriented to the hospital together.

The next day we were divided into three groups. My group was oriented to our floor (State II). It happened to be an open ward for women. What a relief to find I wasn't assigned to a locked ward. I had a feeling that the violent ones would pick up the scent of fear on me.

Our class and clinical hours never added up to more than eight in a day. No evening or night shifts. Amazing! Most of the work schedules are from 7 A.M. to noon. Class was from 1 P.M. to 3 P.M. Sometimes work was 7-11, and class 11-3. We never worked past 9:30 at night.

We all decided to get a perfect suntan while we're in Galveston. We hit the beach on April 4th and started with just a few minutes of sun. Everyone coordinated and counted the time on each side— turning over in unison. So dedicated were we that we sunned on the tar roof of the dorm if we didn't have time for the beach.

It didn't take us long to meet some of the medical students. We were living near the frat houses. The parties were mostly drunken bores. Few of us made a habit of the parties or the med Students— the times we did were usually disasters. Some of us did hang out at the Phi Chi house. We became friends with a few of the guys, and we liked the pool.

Carol, being a rich married lady, owned a television set. Whoever was in the dorm at night sat on the floor in her room to watch late movies. There was a movie every night on one channel called "Late Date Movie." We liked the crazy guy who had a running patter during commercial breaks.

It's amazing. The food is even good. We have a choice between two cafeterias on campus. We can also use food tickets in the hospital drug store—they make a terrific club sandwich—and a banana split to die for.

By mid May Peggy was winning hands down with the tan. We were all working diligently though. We were on the beach at least several times a week. One day Peggy, Joyce, and I were doing our turn over and I stepped on my swimsuit strap—stripping my suit to my waist. The beach was full of people. No one applauded!

I'm beginning to feel that I know Rusty Altizer well enough to marry him myself. He's a constant topic in late night conversations with Joyce. His personality seems to permeate our room.

One fateful night of partying at the Phi Chi pool gave us something to remember. We picked up a stray kitten that was hanging around the psych buildings and took it back to the dorm. Carol bathed it in a sink. Then we got the idea to take it along to the party. All of us cat lovers let the kitten crawl all over us as we sat by the pool in our swim suits. Girls from other affiliating schools were at the party. In a few days many of us started noticing itchy red places on different parts of our bodies. Student health doctors had no idea what they were—even though there seemed to be an epidemic among students from several nursing schools. I happened to mention it to one of the staff psychiatrists one day at work. He looked at the three on my shoulder (they were my only ones) and said, "if you go in one of the vacant rooms and take off your clothes, I can tell you what they are". After he received the anticipated chortles from his audience of medical students and nurses, he told me that it was plain old ringworm. We lined up at student health and were issued medication. Peggy and Dottie had so many ringworms that pictures were taken to send to a medical journal. I think the count was over a hundred on Peggy's legs alone.

On May 12th, Ruthie, Shirley, and I went out with Robert while Joni was working. We all started crying in our "several" beers over our love life—except Robert—he was just consoling us (and drinking beer). We went to several places (including our favorite—the Cave). When we went back to Joni's apartment she was waiting with fire in her eyes. Robert prudently straggled behind and then skipped out. We all spent ages looking for him. Even Ed and Curtis (who were visiting), drove around to try to find him. He finally appeared out of the blue—sauntering up the drive eating an ice cream cone—innocence personified.

We went to an A.A. meeting this evening as part of class. I guess you had to be an alcoholic to get something out of it. Our biggest reaction was queasiness at listening to their personal tales of woe. Several of us felt an urgent need for a beer after.

All of us had a two week tour of working in the treatment rooms. It was interesting, but rather disturbing. Rows and rows of people in different stages of insulin shock really did look like a snake pit—or a torture chamber. No less grotesque was the routine that was used to terminate the DSI. A nurse and doctor walked along by the beds with a rolling cart filled with syringes of 50% glucose. They had to very quickly find a vein and inject the patient before the insulin did permanent damage. Sometimes there was blood all over the beds from the puncture wound left by the large bore needle and the lack of time to apply pressure. It usually became the students' lot to clean up and calm the patients. Then we had to convince them to drink a large glass of sweetened orange juice and get them into breakfast. Not always an easy task! One day a young man that had just had his orange juice ran straight at the plate glass window and went through it. He continued to run, and it took a long time for the orderlies to catch him. I can't imagine how he avoided it, but he wasn't injured seriously.

The electric shock room was even worse. I hated when the patients received the jolt of Anectine and couldn't breathe in the seconds before the current hit their brain. They always remembered that feeling afterward also. The convulsions during the treatment didn't look therapeutic to me. One of my patients died during electric shock treatment. Luckily I wasn't in the treatment room that day.

On May 17th Don Flewell, Jack Ritter, and Jess Smelly came to visit. Ruthie and I went out with them, and drove all over the island. The guys were in Houston for a military parade. The next day my sister came to Galveston and picked Dottie and me up to go to watch the festivities. We waited at the end of the parade route for Don, Jack, and Jess, and then went to an air show at Ellington Field. They returned us to Galveston after. (Poor Ruthie was working.)

A group of us walked all the way to the Boliver Ferry crossing (barefoot), then rode across to Boliver Island on the ferry. It seemed like a great adventure. We didn't even get off—just rode back.

The patients will even sometimes allow us to take them for long walks—if we beg (they may have caught on that we wanted to get out more than they did). My group shopped in Woolworth's one day—explored the Strand—and steered clear of the bars (since a few of the patients seemed far too interested in the first couple we passed). Most of the time our strolls were in the beach area.

Some of the patients played cards in the dining room of family housing with the student nurses. I assume this could be considered therapy—according to who they were playing against.

It's hard to get used to this being "work." We spend most of our time talking to patients. We're even encouraged to sit down with them. They're expected to bathe themselves and make their own beds. (There are maids who make the beds if necessary.) We do give the medications and a do a few nursing procedures, but it's a far cry from the very physical hospital chores of our previous experience.

Lou and I were ejected from the medical library on May 24th. We were supposed to be working on a class assignment. For some reason we started laughing and couldn't stop. The librarians didn't appreciate the humor—specially when it escalated to hysterics.

A medical student buddy took a group of us through the anatomy lab one night. We had to do it in the dark since no one actually gave us permission. So we used a flashlight to look at the cadavers, but couldn't find the nerve to lift the plastic cover and look at the same time. One person would lift the cover with her eyes averted, while the others peered in the vats. The cadavers were all blackened and mummified from preserving solution. Shelves, brimming with bottles of body parts, lined all the walls. The med student finished the tour by telling us tales of how they prepared the cadavers by hanging them from hooks with ice tongs in their ears while injecting blue dye in the veins and red in the arteries for further dissection and study. (Made those frogs we worked on seem pretty tame.)

We, of course, had classes, and worked, with the other affiliates. We became friends with some of the Methodist students from Dallas and Baptist students from Houston. Strangely enough, we didn't get to know any of the Prairie View students. It was a different group from the ones in Houston. My only time to ever skip a class in nursing school was with Miss Bynum, a Baptist student. She had a car and was driving to Houston for the week-end (and just had to leave early!). I went along to get the bus to my parents' house. I was scared to death I would be caught. It felt like I was committing a mortal sin—and probably was.

We finished work at John Sealy on June 21st. Johnny Stroud picked a group of us up to drive back to Temple. It was about 110 degrees in the shade and Johnny was driving a car whose heater wouldn't turn off. We were dressed in shorts and looked frazzled and bedraggled. Johnny stopped to get gas along the highway and we all piled out to get a coke. The gas station operator asked where we were coming from. When we told him that we just left Galveston—he said, "I've heard they're making it difficult for you there lately." (There was a recent crackdown on prostitution.)

We moved back in the dorm in Temple on June 22nd. The next day (Sunday) we had a picnic at Belton Lake to celebrate our return. Jerry Janes joined us, and even behaved!

It was so hot in the dorm that we had to sit in front of the little oscillating fans to get enough breeze to apply our makeup. (Of course there was still no air conditioning, and it was hard to readjust.) The starched uniforms were very uncomfortable in the heat. Carol was fond of lining the back of her collar with Kleenex to cut down on chafing. Once she tried a sanitary napkin in place of the Kleenex. I don't recall if she actually wore it to work.

We started sleeping on the upstairs porch most nights to keep cool—pulling our mattresses out after dark, and back in early in the mornings. I don't know how many times we were entertainment for the patients or doctors on the upper floors of the clinic when we didn't wake up in time. The sun came up early and sometimes we had to crawl so we couldn't be seen from the street (panties being our only attire). Gladys threatened to tell on us, but didn't, of course. Neither did anyone else—or Miss Cole would have put an end to it--and probably us in the process.

The dorm had a fire escape (of sorts) from the second floor. There was no door—access was through a low window. The stairs were used mostly to hang the mops to dry. Dot and I did go down the fire escape one night to dodge dates that were coming to the front door. We had neglected to tell them we had made plans with some-one else.

Went over to see Joyce's wedding gown. It's already finished and hanging on the back of a closet door at her parents' home.

It seems strange to not have classes. Our work schedule is enough to keep us off the streets though.

While working on II West some of us were assigned to go in at 6 A.M. to do morning care. One night that I worked 11-7 we had a death in the early morning hours. The family had been called and we were waiting for them (and the hearse) to arrive (we had no morgue). I had been sitting in the room with the patient, but left for a moment. Frenchie was the one to arrive at 6 a.m. She dutifully gave the dead lady a wet wash cloth and cranked her bed up—then went on to the next patient. (Frenchie said later that she just thought the lady wasn't very friendly.)

We spent a lot of time in Joni and Robert's apartment. It had air conditioning, was conveniently close to the dorm, and often had food in the refrigerator.

On July 3rd Lou had a date with Bill Conn. She asked Frenchie and me to go out with them and two of Bill's friends. I have no idea who my date was, but I took one look at him and "accidentally" got in the car next to Harry Wharton, who was supposed to be Frenchie's date. Harry wasn't really that great either, but his car was—a turquoise '57 Chevrolet! I later made a sundress to match the color.

I started working on pediatrics on July 7th with Miss Miertschen and Mrs. Rhodes. Frenchie and I were both assigned there, but rarely worked together. I developed severe laryngitis and didn't want to go see Dr. Hammond. Frenchie gave me a daily injection of penicillin for several days as we changed shifts (obviously at times the RN's weren't around). I couldn't talk at all during the siege. A welcome respite for everyone in the dorm!

I learned one thing from working in pediatrics. It won't be my chosen specialty. Scott and White is certainly less stressful than Jeff Davis, but still quite physically and mentally tiring. And this unit is strange—all the patients are in one large room, with the nurses station in the middle—there is never a moment away from the kids.

One of the pediatricians had a pet procedure to hydrate children with severe diarrhea. He *very very* slowly infused IV solution sub-cutaneously, with needles in each thigh on a Y tubing. It was the absolute worst thing to watch and control. If it infused too rapidly the tissues would be swollen and damaged. If too slow the needles clogged with blood.

We didn't get out of having physical exams by nearing graduation. In a bad case of senioritis, several of us decided that we couldn't be bothered with urinating in our specimen bottles. We delegated that to some of the "all too willing to please" freshman girls. My fresh-man turned out to have albumin in her urine. I was swiftly sent over to the emergency room where a student practiced her catheteri-zation procedure on me.

We became quite fond of some of the freshman girls living in our dorm—even managed to live with Sylvia's frequent high pitched screams.

Andy was now seriously dating, and her boyfriend was kind (or foolish) enough to loan us his truck to drive around once in a while. Hopefully, he didn't follow us!

Lou, Ruthie, and I visited Don Flewell in the hospital at Fort Hood on July 19th. His surgery was simple, but painful, and in an area that assured no one would ask to see his "scar."

A school tradition that we really enjoyed was the dinner at Stage-coach Inn for graduating seniors. We sat in the courtyard under an enormous old oak tree. Very impressive!

The graduation uniforms are here. No one likes the length, but we've been told that we can't change them, they must all be 13 inches from the floor. The uniforms are great otherwise.

On a week-end trip home (so no one could see) I hemmed my uniform to the length I deemed most becoming to me! Narcissism wins over conformity, and selfishness rules!

Worked my last shift (3-11 on pediatrics) as a student nurse—with mixed feelings. I was excited knowing I would soon be stepping into a whole new world, and sad to leave behind the life I had come to love.

Made a trip to Rogers to the liquor store for supplies. We've decided to have champagne and vodka for our post graduation party. Bought stemmed glasses to serve the wine in style.

Butterflies. Anxiety. Anticipation. Unbridled joy. August 17th found us in mad dashes in and out of the dorm as we shuttled between our guests, last minute packing, party preparation, hair-do's, and getting dressed for graduation.

How professional we all look. The uniforms are perfect. (No one noticed that mine is the shortest one.) The black stripe on the caps--the crowning glory.

The actual graduation ceremony seemed to pass in a blur. There were speakers; I hardly listened. At the end Miss Cole pinned each of us as our name was called. Those lovely stars were ours for a few shining moments—then Miss Gallman was waiting in the wings to reclaim them. We won't see them again until we pass state boards.

A quick trip back to the dorm to change, and we're on to the Shangri-La. How fitting that our last hours are spent there. The owners of the Shangri-La agreed to let us bring in our own drinks—since they served only beer. They chilled the champagne and glasses for us ahead of time. It must have been a going away gift to us, since I'm sure they didn't make any money from our party. They set up a long table, big enough for us to all sit together, and seemed to happily put up with all the noise. Champagne flowed along with a few tears and a lot of laughter. It's hard to believe that most of us are going our separate ways after tonight.

I spent the latter part of the night in the dorm—sleeping in a bed no longer mine. My chariot (in the form of my sister's car) arrived at the break of dawn to transport me away from Temple. I looked back as we drove out of sight. The campus was empty and still. So was my heart.

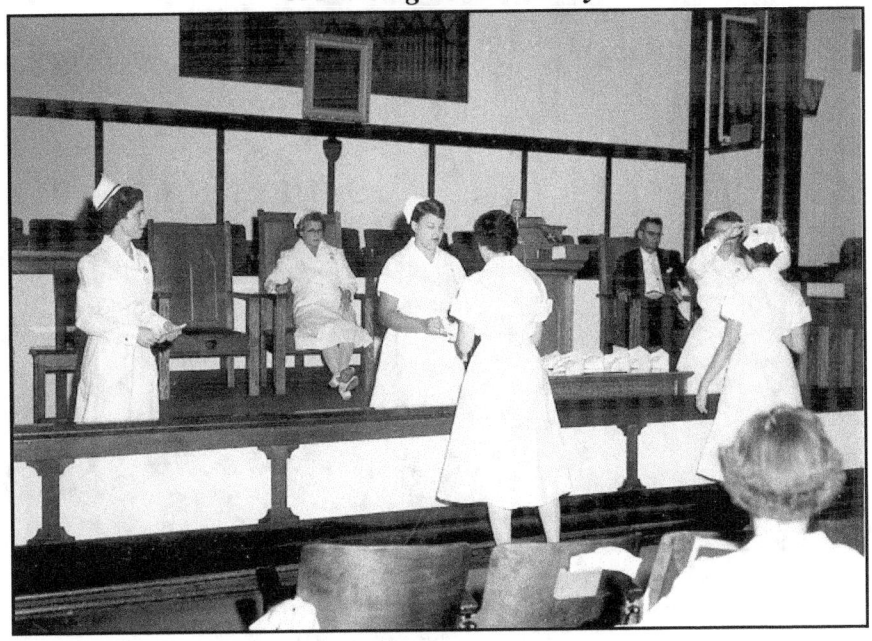

Capping ceremony
Miss Gallman, Miss Cole, Miss Bohls
Marion Zacharias presenting caps
Joyce Helbert and Norma Hammond receiving caps.

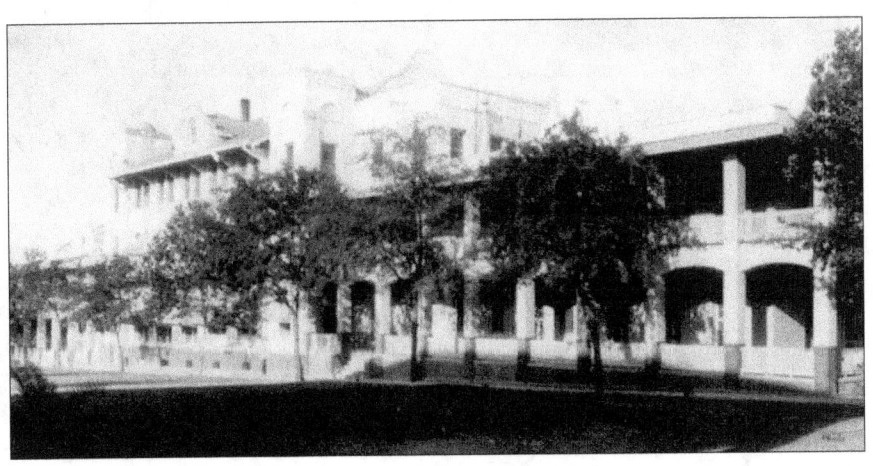

Main building - Scott & White Hospital, Temple, Texas

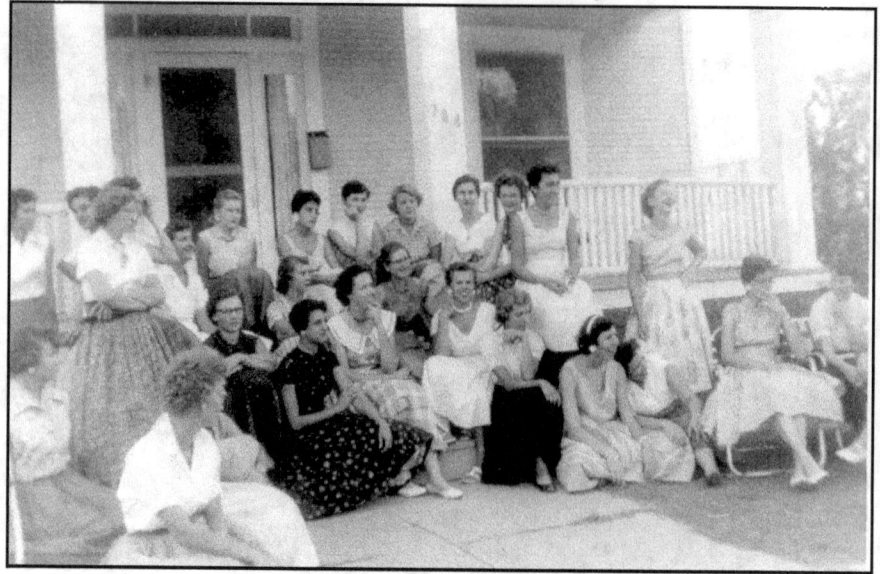

Front porch gathering of student nurses
Senior Dorm

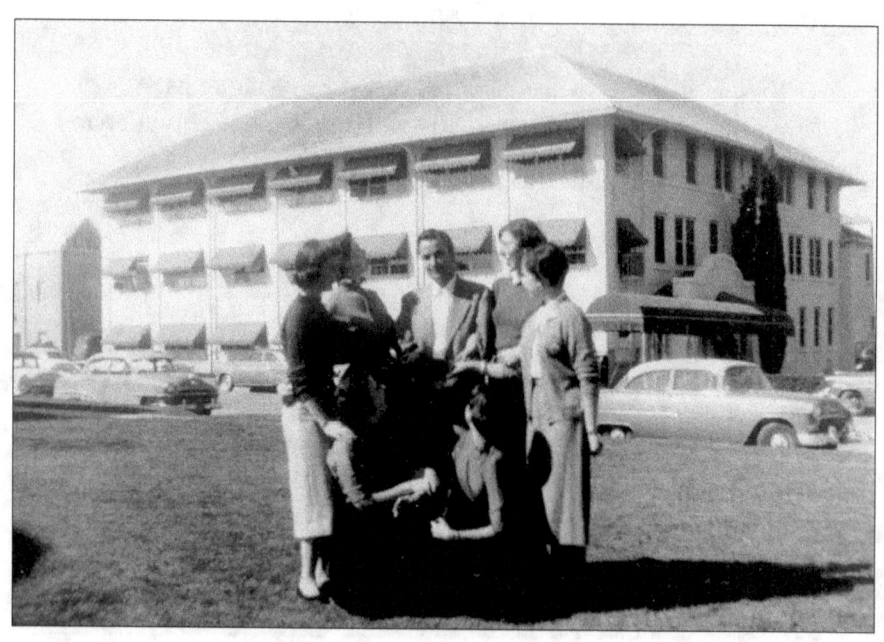

In front of Scott & White Clinic

In front of Scott & White Clinic

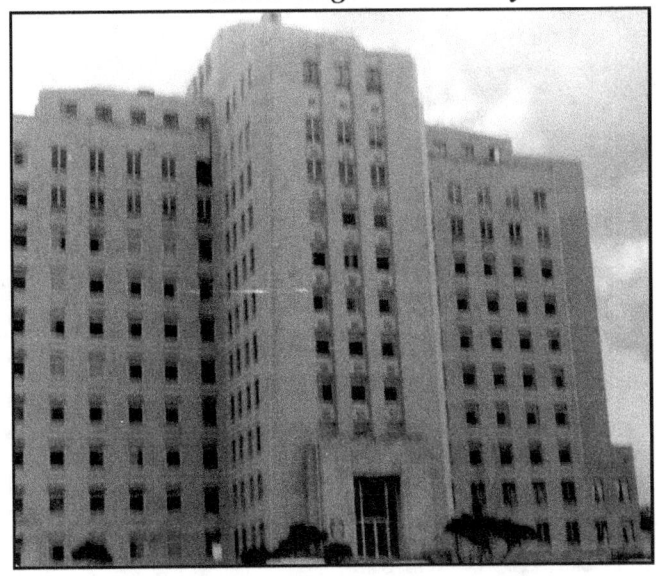

Jefferson Davis Hospital
Houston, Texas

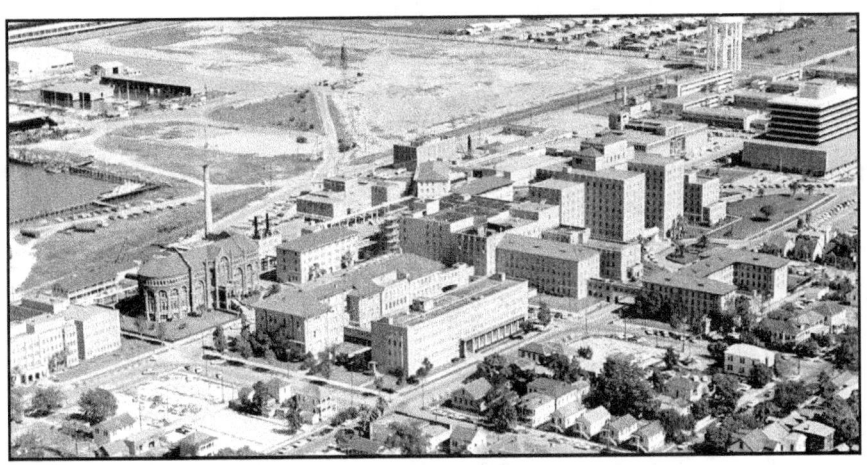

John Sealy Hospital
University of Texas-Medical Branch
Galveston, Texas

Commencement Exercises

of the

School of Nursing

of

Scott and White Memorial Hospital

CLASS OF NINETEEN HUNDRED FIFTY-SEVEN

Christ Episcopal Church

SATURDAY EVENING, AUGUST 17, 1957 AT 7:30 O'CLOCK

Program

Processional	MR. MARVIN TARRANT
Invocation	REV. J. B. DOBBINS
Solo	MR. JOE SCARCELLA III
Introduction of Speaker	MR. W. E. ARNOLD
Class Address	MR. E. M. COLLIER
Presentation of Maud Scott Award	MR. JAMES HARRIS SCOTT
Presentation of Class	MISS LAVERNE GALLMAN
Awarding of Diplomas	P. M. BASSEL, M. D., *Chairman of the Board*
Awarding of Pins	MISS ANNA LAURA COLE, *Director of Nurses*
School Song	STUDENTS
Benediction	REV. J. B. DOBBINS
Recessional	MR. MARVIN TARRANT

Reception in Parish House

Class of 1957

ILA CAROL BLEDSOE BALL

JOAN JONES DAVENPORT

MARJORIE ROWE DEES

LOUINE FRANC DOLAN

FRANCES ANN FRENCH

NORMA GENE HAMMOND

ANNA JOYCE HELBERT

ERMA LARUTH HOGAN

JANICE DRAKE JACKSON

PEGGY SUE LOGAN

DOROTHEA NELL STROUD

SAMUELLA SUE STUTTS

AMOR TIBI

We're proud to be a part of
the girls who serve in white

We're also proud that we are
a part of Scott and White

We'll strive to keep her standards
of serving all mankind

We pledge our hearts, our lives, our all
to keep our goal in mind-

Here's glory to our school
of dear ole' Scott and White

We shall forever serve her
with courage, hope and might

We'll try to make her pleased with
our work, our daily lives

We'll try to make her proud of
her graduates as years go by.

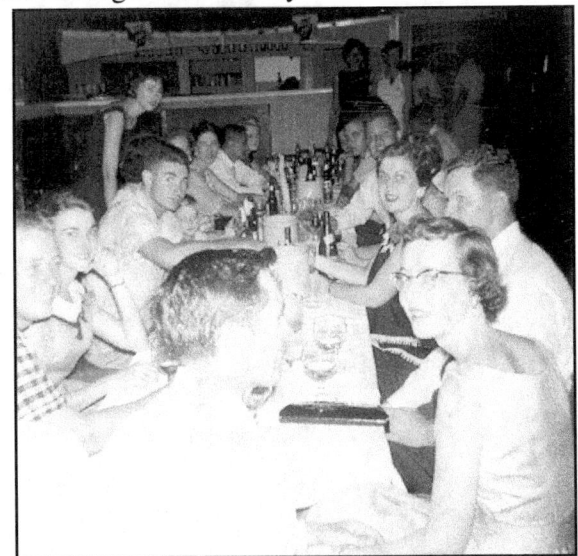

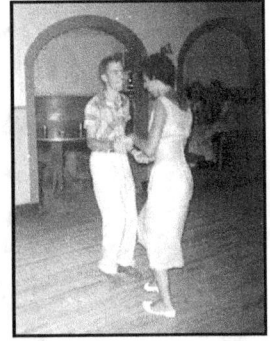

Graduation Night at the Shangri-La

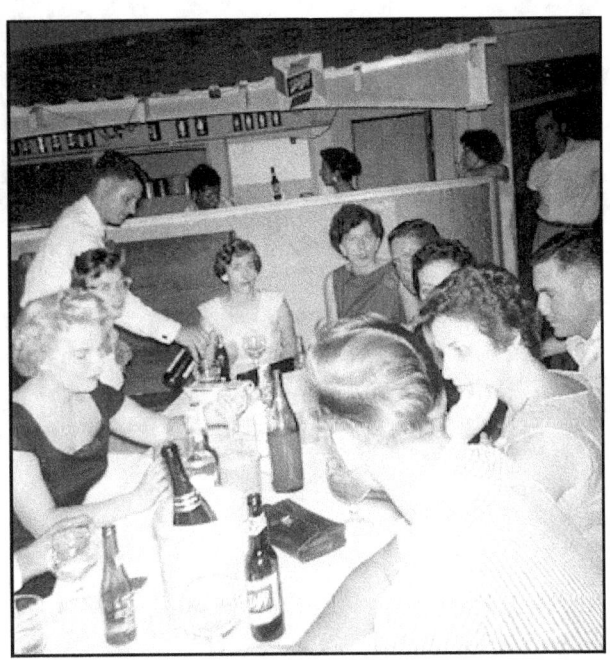

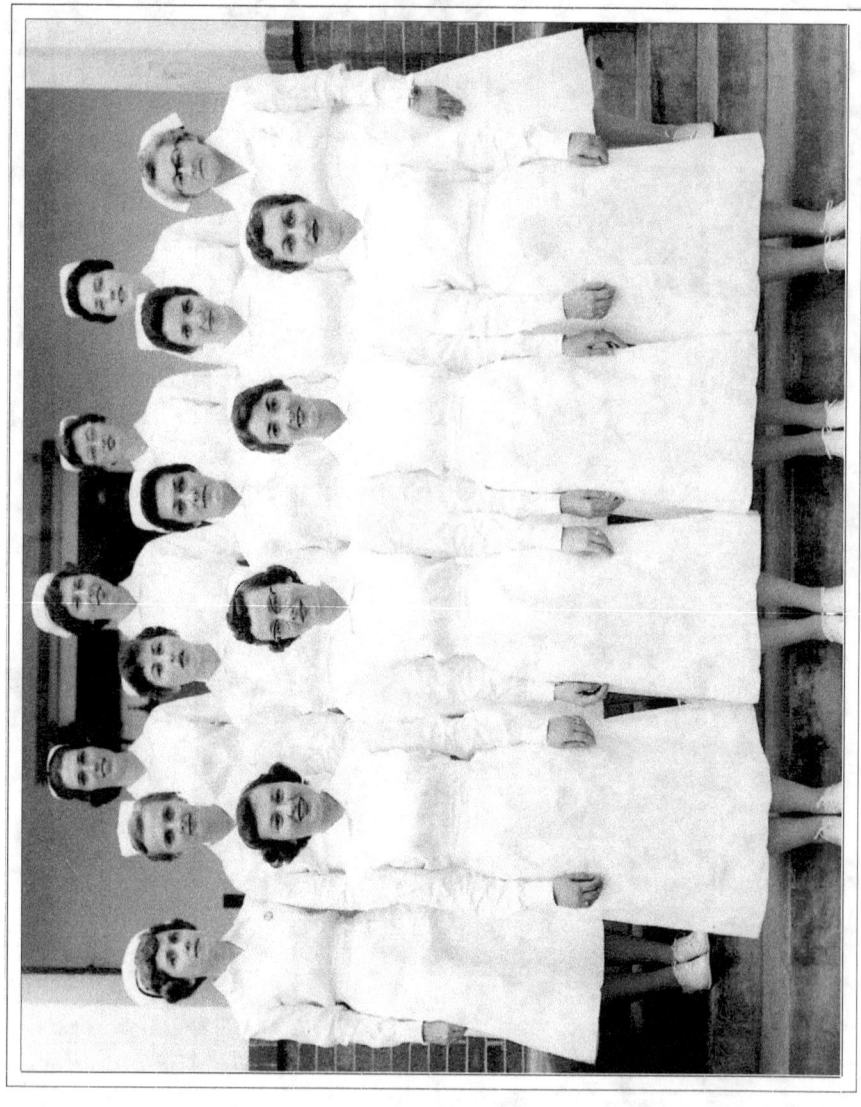

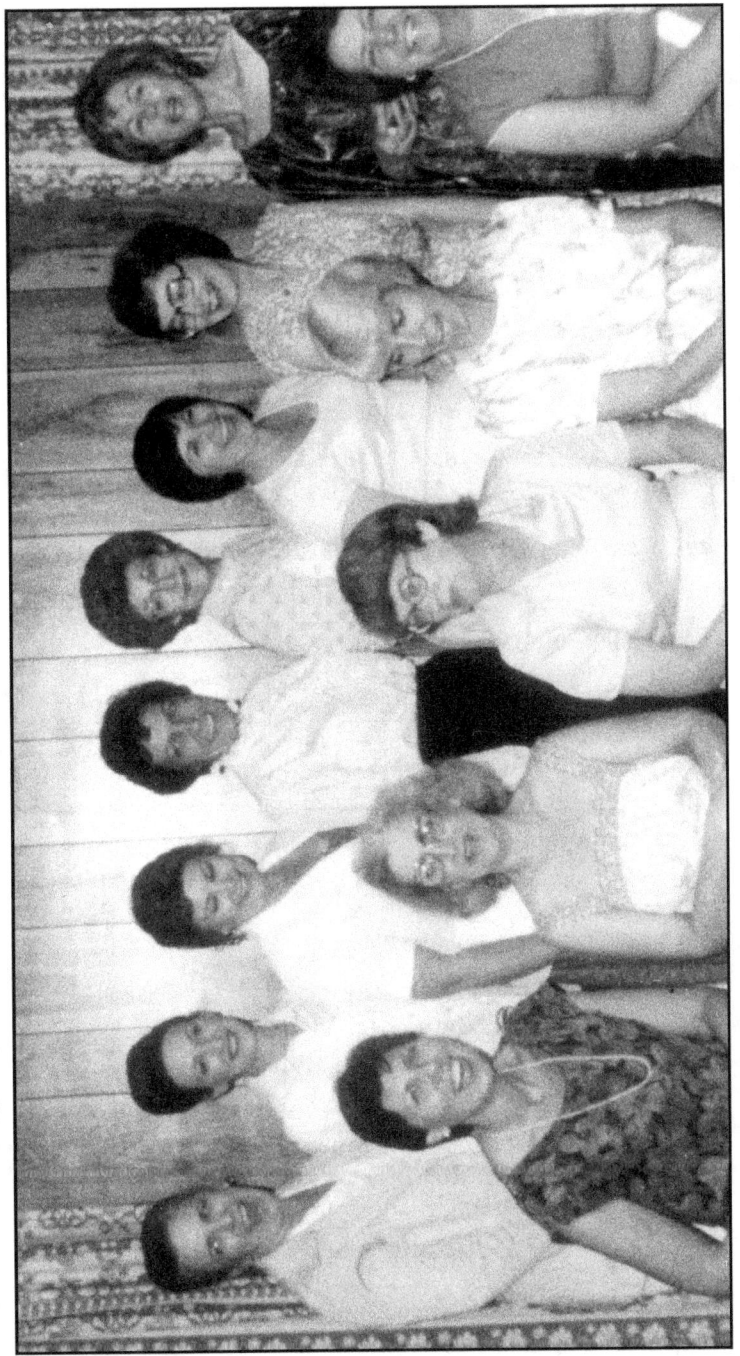

From left rear: Frances French Daigle, Louine Dolan Graham, Shirley Roberts Holleman, Peggy Logan Baechtle, Muriel Holmes Clarke, Marjorie Rowe Harris, Joan Jones Davenport, Norma Hammond McLoughlin, Dorothea Stroud Hart, Carol Bledsoe Ball, Ruthie Hogan Flewell, Samuella Stutts Martin, Joyce Helbert Altizer

25th Year Reunion

Norma Hammond McLoughlin grew up in Polk County, Texas, and graduated from Big Sandy High School. She then graduated from Scott and White Memorial Hospital School of Nursing in Temple, Texas, and later worked as an RN in a wide variety of nursing fields before becoming a school nurse in a private school in New Orleans. She returned to Texas to work in neonatal care before retiring. She has also written *Camp Ruby...A Place in Time, Sawdust Memories* (a history of Camden, Texas), *Leggett, Texas....Its History and People, Footsteps in the Sands of Time (*a history of the Hammond family) and *Deep Roots in the Tall Pines* (a history of southeast Polk County, Texas).

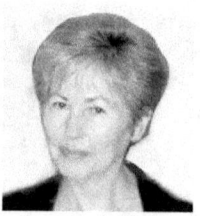

Norma Hammond McLoughlin
155 Rush Haven Dr.
The Woodlands, Texas 77381

281 367-3147
mclou@hal-pc.org
JNMclou@gmail.com